Rest

'A game-changing book for the weary modern world'
Brigid Schulte, author of *Overwhelmed*

'I loved *Rest*. It places rest back on the pedestal it so clearly deserves and generously points out – through great stories and acute insight – things to reflect on and build into our own lives'
Rohan Gunatillake, founder of Mindfulness Everywhere and creator of the bestselling buddhify app

'Good books are interesting and valuable; but the best books reframe the way you see the world, getting you thinking differently about everyday situations and assumptions. *Rest* does just that. With a fascinating combination of research and historical examples, your view of rest – as what you do when you are not working – is turned upside down. A thoroughly enjoyable, insightful and life-enhancing book'
Tony Crabbe, international business psychologist

'In his fascinating, well-researched and highly readable new book, Dr Pang makes an excellent case for the critical importance of rest in our lives. You will consider how and why you rest in a completely new light after reading this book'
Wendy Suzuki, professor of neural science and psychology, New York University, and author of *Healthy Brain, Happy Life*

'Want to be creative and get more done? A new paradigm of work is emerging and this fascinating book will be an indispensable guide'
Peter Fleming, author of *The Mythology of Work*

'It's high noon for the global economy's thinking class, who are locked in a losing battle for clarity in a crowded, clickable world. This book is a science-packed call to arms: it's time to claim rest as a right and pay close attention to the needs of our beleaguered brains'
Anthony T

ABOUT THE AUTHOR

Alex Soojung-Kim Pang is the founder of the Restful Company, a consulting company in Silicon Valley, California, and a visiting academic at Stanford University. He is the author of *The Distraction Addiction* and has written for *Slate*, *Wired*, *Atlantic Monthly* and *Scientific American*. He lives in Silicon Valley.

@rest_book

www.deliberate.rest

Rest

Why You Get More Done

When You Work Less

ALEX SOOJUNG-KIM PANG

PENGUIN LIFE

AN IMPRINT OF

PENGUIN BOOKS

PENGUIN LIFE

UK | USA | Canada | Ireland | Australia
India | New Zealand | South Africa

Penguin Life is part of the Penguin Random House group of companies
whose addresses can be found at global.penguinrandomhouse.com

 Penguin
Random House
UK

First published in the United States of America by Basic Books, an imprint of Perseus Books,
a division of PBG Publishing, LLC, a subsidiary of Hachette Book Group, Inc. 2016
First published in Great Britain by Penguin Life 2017
001

Printed in Great Britain by Clays Ltd, St Ives plc

A CIP catalogue record for this book is available from the British Library

ISBN: 978–0–241–21728–3

www.greenpenguin.co.uk

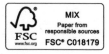 MIX
Paper from
responsible sources
FSC® C018179

Penguin Random House is committed to a
sustainable future for our business, our readers
and our planet. This book is made from Forest
Stewardship Council® certified paper.

For Thomas Parke Hughes and Linda Wiedmann

Contents

Contents

Introduction

THIS IS A BOOK about work. It is also, of course, a book about rest. This sounds paradoxical, but it illustrates the book's central idea.

Many of us are interested in how to work better, but we don't think very much about how to rest better. Productivity books offer life hacks, advice about how to get more done, or stories about what CEOs or famous writers do. But they say almost nothing about the role of rest in the lives or careers of creative, productive people. When they do mention rest, they tend to treat it as nothing more than a physical necessity or inconvenience.

Books about rest or leisure, meanwhile, seem mainly interested in escaping work, not improving your ability to do meaningful work. They praise idleness as an antidote to overwork and an expression of wisdom. The clever man may work smarter, not harder, they say, but the creative man doesn't work at all. Other writers portray leisure as a luxury to be consumed and broadcast. For them, the good life is an endless summer, shared with just the right washed-out Instagram filter.

As a result, we see work and rest as binaries. Even more problematic, we think of rest as simply the absence of work, not as something that stands on its own or has its own qualities. Rest is merely a negative space in a life defined by toil and ambition and accomplishment. When we define ourselves by our work, by our dedication and effectiveness and willingness to go the extra mile, then it's easy to see rest as the negation of all those things. If your work is your self, when you cease to work, you cease to exist.

When we think of rest as work's opposite, we take it less seriously and even avoid it. Americans work more and vacation less than almost any other nationality in the world. Contrary to the expectations of economists (and in defiance of common sense), as we become more productive, we work longer hours, not shorter. We leave vacation days unused. When we do finally go on vacation, we compulsively check our e-mail.

I argue that we misunderstand the relationship between work and rest. Work and rest are not polar opposites. You cannot talk about rest without also talking about work. Writing about only one is like writing a romance and naming only one of the lovers. Rest is not work's adversary. Rest is work's partner. They complement and complete each other.

Further, you cannot work well without resting well. Some of history's most creative people, people whose achievements in art and science and literature are legendary, took rest very seriously. They found that in order to realize their ambitions, to do the kind of work they wanted to, they needed rest. The right kinds of rest would restore their energy while allowing their muse, that mysterious part of their minds that helps drive the creative process, to keep going.

So work and rest aren't opposites like black and white or good and evil; they're more like different points on life's wave. You can't have a crest without a trough. You can't have the highs without the lows. Neither can exist without the other.

We underestimate how much good serious rest can do us. And we also underestimate how much we can do if we take rest seriously.

I enjoy both good work and good rest. I love intellectual and physical challenges, the sense of purpose and accomplishment that comes from getting both big and little things done. For me, the feeling that accompanies a creative breakthrough—and even just the feeling of chasing an idea, immersing myself in a problem, and matching my talents against a big challenge—is as addicting and exciting as any game, as physically satisfying and stimulating as food (and I really like food), as emotionally fulfilling and essential as being in love. Hard work can be both honorable and rewarding. I look back fondly on some of my hardest jobs because of the camaraderie I found working long hours with good people, pushing the boundaries of our company, and trying new things. I find visions of the "good life" that feature wealth-creation systems and early retirement crass and distasteful. In contrast, the arguments of psychologists like Viktor Frankl and Mihaly Csikszentmihalyi that the good life is defined by a search for meaning and an abundance of challenges, make profound intuitive sense.

So my interest in rest doesn't arise from a distaste for work. It starts with a sense that we should embrace challenges, not avoid them; that work isn't a bad thing but an absolute necessity for a meaningful, fulfilling life. But I've also come to see our respect for overwork as, perhaps a bit paradoxically, intellectually lazy. Measuring time is literally the easiest way to assess someone's dedication and productivity, but it's also very unreliable.

At the same time, I love serious rest. Not idle hours watching Russian dashboard cam videos and taking Facebook quizzes to see which *Twilight* character I am, but beautifully empty hours that stretch out, untouchable by clients or colleagues or (especially) children. I love sleeping, the physical sensation of my body settling into bed, of unconsciousness rising like the moon. I'm motivated to finish my work by the prospect of an hour at the gym.

Of course, I can't claim any special insight here. The ancient Greeks saw rest as a great gift, as the pinnacle of civilized life. The Roman Stoics argued that you cannot have a good life without good work. Indeed, virtually every ancient society, recognized that both work and rest were necessary for a good life: one provided the means to live, the other gave meaning to life. Today, we've lost touch with that wisdom, and our lives are poorer and less fulfilling as a result. It's time we rediscovered the good that rest can do.

WHILE I'VE HAD an interest in the psychology of creativity since college, I only began thinking seriously about the role of rest in creative lives more recently—specifically, during a winter evening I spent with my wife at a café in Cambridge, England. I was a visiting fellow at Microsoft Research, working on a project that eventually turned into my book *The Distraction Addiction*. We would often go to one of the town's many cafés or pubs after dinner. On this evening, we settled at a table with a stack of articles and two books I was reading: Virginia Woolf's *A Room of One's Own* and John Kay's *Obliquity*.

In *A Room of One's Own*, Woolf compares the lives of dons at well-endowed ancient colleges and the pinched existence of faculty at the newer women's colleges. The ancient colleges offered far greater opportunities to excel, according to Woolf, not because of their richer endowments but because of their more leisurely pace: generous research budgets and obliging staffs gave faculty time for long walks and lengthy conversations. Meanwhile, in *Obliquity* John Kay observes that companies that flourished when they focused on great work and customer service often stumble when new executive teams institute strategies focused on improving financial performance. Companies that put profits first, Kay argues, are more likely to lose money than those that treat profit as a by-product of doing great work.

These two books triggered an insight about a third that I had been carrying around like a good luck charm, hoping that some of the success the author enjoyed during his time in Cambridge might rub off on me: *The Double Helix*, James

Watson's account of his and Francis Crick's discovery of the structure of DNA. Usually I focused on the competition and conflict in the story, but Wolff's argument that leisure enables productivity and Kay's idea of obliquity made me aware of something I'd never paid much attention to. Watson and Crick didn't just spend time hunkered down in the lab. Lots of the action happened over long lunches at the Eagle pub, during afternoon walks around Cambridge, or while browsing in bookstores. And Watson, despite being locked in a race against some of the most brilliant scientific minds of the century, was constantly running off to conferences, going on vacation in the Alps, or playing tennis. One of his contemporaries said that Watson had time for girls and tennis because he was a genius. But Woolf and Kay made me think: Maybe he was a genius because he made time for girls and tennis. Maybe creative achievement needs to be approached obliquely.

This idea lay in the back of my mind through the winter. My wife and I both worked hard and got a lot done during our sabbatical, but we also found time for evenings in the pub, Sunday walks to the Orchard, quick trips to London, and weekends in Edinburgh and Bath and Oxford. It was an intense and productive time, yet also oddly unhurried. As ardent Anglophiles, we found being in Cambridge intellectually energizing. But I began to wonder if our productivity had as much to do with pace of our lives as the place we lived. I started to think that maybe our familiar ways of working and living and our unquestioned assumptions about the need to stay always connected, to keep one eye on the inbox at the playground or the dinner table, to treat weekends as a time to catch up on work, and to hold vacations in contempt, actually don't work as well as we think.

A survey of the lives of contemporary leaders and creatives made clear that I'd have to cast my net wider to understand rest in productive lives. With a few notable exceptions, today's leaders treat stress and overwork as a badge of honor, brag about how little they sleep and how few vacations days they take, and have their reputations as workaholics carefully tended by publicists and corporate PR firms. They remind us how the working lives of even the most powerful people unfold in an environment saturated with unquestioned assumptions about the virtue and inescapable necessity of constant work. Whether we embrace the idea that overwork is essential for productivity and creativity or reject it, we all are defined by it.

When I looked to the past, though, the life I had lived during my sabbatical resurfaced. In previous centuries, leading authors, scientists, politicians, and businessmen created masterpieces, won elections, and captained industries while finding ample time for long walks and regular naps, weekends away, even weeks-long vacations. Many had been hard-charging workaholics in their youth, but while their ambitions never flagged, as they matured they learned to lean back, develop sustainable routines, and make rest an essential part of their creative lives. They had to learn to rest, to pay close attention to how they worked and what worked for them. They became sensitive to how changes in their routine affected their ability to think. They experimented with their schedules to discover when they had the most energy and focus, and they tweaked their habits to find rhythms and rituals that helped them stay on their game. In other words, they were not all figures perched on the border between genius and madness, driven to create by unconscious compulsion and uncontrollable passion. They were more like athletes constantly searching for a new workout, improved pregame routine, or energizing diet that would give them an edge.

Anyone looking to the past for models of how to better balance work and rest must deal with the objection that previous eras are too different from our own to allow for useful comparisons. Life was simpler a century ago, distractions were fewer, economies were more forgiving, and leisure was respected. People had more time for rest. Today, the competing demands of work and home, of colleagues and children, leave us with no time to ourselves. Technologies that promised to make our work more flexible instead chain us to work and create the expectation that we'll always be accessible to clients, colleagues, and children. A perpetually uncertain economy requires us to accept these terms or be replaced. In a twenty-four/seven, always-on world, the concept of turning off is an anachronism.

But if our ancestors had more time to rest, nobody told them. A hundred fifty years ago, the Victorians were keenly aware of living through an era of rapid globalization and economic growth, scientific and technological revolutions, massive social changes, and new kinds of threats from terrorists and ideologies. The railroad, telegraph, and steam engine brought the world closer together, boosted economic productivity and trade, and allowed news to travel the world at fantastic speeds. But technologies were also destroying local habits, upending the traditional rhythms of village and country life, and intruding on peace and quiet. Nineteenth-century doctors worried that the fast pace of urban life and speed of railroads were too much for the human brain and that nervous disorders would become epidemic. Labor unions and capitalists battled over working hours and the pace of factory work. And reformers and psychologists warned about the dangers of overwork.

Consider William James's diagnosis of overwork in his 1899 essay "Gospel of Relaxation." He argued that Americans had become accustomed to overwork, to living with an "inner panting and expectancy" and bringing "breathlessness and tension" to work. Americans wore stress and overwork like fancy jewelry: they internalized bad habits "caught from the social atmosphere, kept up by tradition, and idealized by many as the admirable way of life." He also pointed out that overwork is counterproductive. If "living excitedly and hurriedly would only enable us to do more," he said, then there "would be some compensation, some excuse, for going on so. But the exact reverse is the case." Later generations of efficiency experts confirmed James's argument. During World War I, industrial engineers discovered that factory workers subjected to long months of overtime were less productive and more prone to costly mistakes and industrial accidents than workers who kept more regular hours. Even soldiers who "in the past" had "sought dissipation, not recreation" during leave could find more wholesome rest through organizations like the YMCA and USO, demonstrating "how essential recreation is to efficiency," American business journalist Bertie Charles Forbes wrote. The experience of the victorious armies, he argued, showed that "how we spend our non-working hours determines very largely how capably or incapably we spend our working hours."

In other words, the world and worries of the Victorians sound very much like our own. Lots of people embraced the challenge of matching the productivity of machines and telegraph networks and tried to work faster for longer hours. They were the rule. Yet some chose to be exceptions, and the choices they made about work and rest helped make them exceptional. Their examples show that we are not condemned by impersonal, global forces to lives of overwork. Other kinds of lives are possible.

Their lives also reveal something else. Rest is not something that the world gives us. It's never been a gift. It's never been something you do when you've finished everything else. If you want rest, you have to take it. You have to resist the lure of busyness, make time for rest, take it seriously, and protect it from a world that is intent on stealing it.

History shows that it is possible for ambitious, hard-charging people in a fast-changing world to succeed and create while crafting lives that seem far more leisurely, balanced, and sane. But is it possible to explain why rest is important and why we see consistent patterns in how creative people rested? It turns out that in the last couple decades, discoveries in sleep research, psychology, neuroscience, organizational behavior, sports medicine, sociology, and other fields have given us a wealth of insight into the unsung but critical role that rest plays in strengthening the brain, enhancing learning, enabling inspiration, and making innovation sustainable. This research doesn't just present a general case for the value of rest; it shows how different kinds of rest interact with work in the course of the day, and over the course of a life. It shows us why some kinds of rest stimulate our creativity while others restore our creative energy. It shows us that restorative daytime naps, insight-generating long walks, vigorous exercise, and lengthy vacations aren't unproductive interruptions; they help creative people do their work.

We need to rethink the relationship between work and rest, acknowledge their intimate connection, and rediscover the role that rest can play in helping us be creative and productive. We shouldn't regard rest as a mere physical necessity to be satisfied grudgingly; we should see it as an opportunity. When we stop and rest properly, we're not paying a tax on creativity. We're investing in it.

There are four big insights that guide my thinking about rest and will be touchpoints as I examine the science of rest, explore how rest allows creative people to do great work, and explain how we can apply insights from science and history to our own lives.

First, **work and rest are partners.**

Rest is an essential component of good work. World-class musicians, Olympic athletes, writers, designers, and other accomplished and creative people alternate daily periods of intense work and concentration with long breaks. For a very long time, inspiration and creativity have been something of a mystery: our desire for creativity has always exceeded our understanding of how it works, why it strikes at some times and not others, and what, if anything, we can do to improve it. We're now a few steps closer to uncovering the cognitive processes that are active during creative moments, to seeing what happens in the brain when insight dawns. We don't understand it all, by any means; the brain and creativity are two of the most complex things ever studied, and there are lots of big questions we still can't answer. But it's clear that the brain's creative work is never done, that even in its resting state the brain is plugging away at problems, examining and tossing out possible answers, looking for novelty. This is a process we can't really control. But by learning to rest better, we can support it, let it work, and take notice when it's found something that deserves our attention.

Second, **rest is active.**

When we think of rest, we usually think of passive activities: a nap, lying in the couch, watching sports on television, or binge-watching a popular TV series. That's one form of rest. But physical activity is more restful than we expect, and mental rest is more active than we realize.

For a surprising number of creative people—including people in professions we usually think of as dominated by nerdy, bookish people who don't see the sun for weeks—strenuous, physically challenging, even life-threatening exercise is an essential part of their routine. Some walk miles every day or spend weekends working in their gardens. Some are always in training for the next marathon; others rock climb or scale mountains. Their idea of rest is more vigorous than our idea of exercise.

So why is this restful? Serious exercise helps keep their bodies operating at their peak, which in turn keeps their minds sharp and gives them the energy to do difficult work. But it often also offers subtler psychological benefits: not just stress relief or a chance to clear their minds, but a way to connect with their own pasts. Many serious thinkers choose activities that reflect childhood interests or cultivate skills they first developed with their parents or older siblings. Such choices are part of a bigger, conscious strategy of building a life in which work, play, labor, and leisure all have their place and are all linked together.

Even apparently passive forms of rest turn out to be more physically active than we expect. When you go to sleep, your brain doesn't switch off. It gets busy consolidating memories, reviewing the day's events, and going over problems you've been working on. You get a glimpse of all this behind-the-scenes activity when you dream, but most of this activity happens without your conscious knowledge, and without your direction. The brain also gets busy clearing away toxins and doing physical maintenance; this is important for preventing degenerative neurological diseases. Sleep scientists can see all this activity during REM sleep, when your brain is spiky with electrical activity. Your brain is just as active when you're awake but zoning out. During those moments when your mind is wandering and it feels like your mind has gone blank, your brain is actually driving at full speed. It's just not bothering to bring your conscious self along.

Third, rest is a skill.

Rest turns out to be like sex or singing or running. Everyone basically knows how to do it, but with a little work and understanding, you can learn to do it a lot better. You can enjoy rest more profoundly and be more refreshed and restored. People don't just become world-class performers through deliberate practice. They also practice what you could call *deliberate rest*. They find rest that is psychologically and physically restorative, but also mentally productive. Deliberate rest helps you recover from the stresses and exhaustion of the day, allows new experiences and lessons to settle in your memory, and gives your subconscious mind space to keep working. It's often in these periods of deliberate rest and apparent leisure—when you're not obviously working, or trying to work—that you can have some of your best ideas.

It may seem counterintuitive that rest is something you have to learn how to do well. What's simpler than rest? What is literally more effortless? The only thing more natural than resting is breathing.

Yes, breathing is natural. That's why learning to control one's breathing is something that virtually everyone doing physically strenuous and mentally challenging work must master. Disciplined breathing is one of the most powerful tools we have to counter stress, fear, and distraction.

Learning to breathe more deeply helps athletes compete harder. It helps soldiers and sailors remain calm in battle. It helps musicians sing with greater control. It enables actors and politicians to project their voices.

Rest is the same. Lots of people treat rest as a completely mindless or passive thing. At the end of the day they head to happy hour; on the weekends they go clubbing; on holiday they travel to tropical countries where it's always happy hour and the clubs are always open. They forget themselves until the next morning's hangover, though their Facebook feeds may provide some embarrassing clues to the previous night's activities. But it's also possible to rest in ways that are chal-lenging and rewarding, that make you happier and healthier and literally make your mind work better.

So yes, rest is natural. That's why learning to rest well is so effective.

Finally, **deliberate rest stimulates and sustains creativity.**

For everyone, work and rest are like night and day: the one cannot happen without the other. For super creative people, though, deliberate rest plays an important but usually unrec-ognized role in their creative lives. Some kinds of deliber-ate rest stimulate creativity. Many notable creatives do their most intense work early in the morning, when their minds are freshest and least prone to distraction. They go on walks or take naps during the day to revive and maintain their en-ergy while allowing their subconscious minds time to wander and explore. They often leave a small task unfinished when they stop work, to make it easier to start the next day. They structure their days to have time for both intense, focused work and downtime. These activities help them to develop more creative solutions to problems and to find those solutions more rapidly and with less effort.

Other kinds of deliberate rest make creativity sustainable. Lots of great writers, scientists, and artists exercise regularly, and some are enthusiastic, accomplished athletes. They show an impressive consistency in habits and hobbies. They balance busy lives with deep play, forms of rest that are psychologically restorative, physically active, and personally meaningful. They renew their creative reserves on sabbaticals, retreats during which they're free to travel, explore new ideas, and cultivate new interests. Even though they love losing themselves in work, they maintain strict boundaries between their work and leisure.

The steadiness and consistency that deliberate rest enforces helps explain why those who discover it have longer creative lives, pursue careers as artists or writers while holding down other jobs, and may even discover completely new interests or produce new works when the rest of us are ready to retire. Today we venerate the child entrepreneur and envy the teenage billionaire. But long creative lives challenge our assumptions that youth is essential for good work, that fast beats deliberate, that reckless energy triumphs over steady experience, that greatness is a race against age and obsolescence.

Lives rich in both work and rest also show that long hours don't guarantee higher productivity in creative industries. In a factory or workshop, it's easy to see who the most productive person is: at the end of the day, you can count the number of pieces they've made. Similarly, in some other professions there are clear measures of productivity: the number of customers helped, patients treated, dollars made, cars repaired. But for those of us who work in teams on complicated, open-ended projects, long hours are an expression of our identity and proof of our seriousness. They don't necessarily make us more productive; they make us look more productive. For bosses, it's an easy way to see who's really committed and who isn't—even if it's a terrible predictor of who's going to be good.

In Silicon Valley, where I live, the reigning assumption is that success is a race against time and obsolescence. If you're not rich by the time you're thirty, before your skills become obsolete and you become too decrepit to work hundred-hour weeks, you never will be.

This is a model that works fabulously well for a tiny number of people. But many more people who work this way burn themselves out, with little to show for it at the end. But people who learn to rest deliberately can ultimately get more done, for longer periods of their lives. Their careers aren't races against time, because they don't have to be.

I should also make clear that when I talk about "work," I don't just mean what you do from nine to five or what you're paid to do. Some of us are lucky enough to have jobs that deserve our best selves, and we can carry the lessons of deliberate rest and creative lives with us to work. But what I'm really interested in is what you might call your life's work. This is the work that gives your life meaning; the work that lets you be your best self and helps you become a better self; the work that is an unparalleled pleasure when it goes well and is worth fighting and sacrificing for when it goes poorly; the work that you are willing to organize your life around. I think we all have this work, and the quality of our lives is determined by how well we are able to do it. Indeed, *Rest* is organized around working days and lives. It first describes routines and daily practices—the early morning start, walks, and naps—then broadens to consider activities that happen at a rhythm of weeks (exercise and deep rest) or months or years (vacations and sabbaticals).

So I don't want to deny the importance of work in our lives. Everything from where we live to when or whether we become parents, whether we have pets and plants, and how wide and active our circles of friends are—these are all shaped by the work we do. The challenge we face when learning to rest better is not to avoid work but to discover how to create a better fit between our work and our rest.

This book also isn't meant to just be a life-hacking manual, nor do I advocate turning rest into a tool for increasing our productivity or value in the marketplace. *Rest* does not present one pattern that everyone should follow. I don't propose a single system because I don't believe that there's a single way we all should work. Workplaces vary hugely in their rhythms and demands, and human brains are too varied, creativity too multifaceted, and lives too diverse for simple recommendations. Still, I do believe that everyone has work that they can do brilliantly; that we all have the potential to find the work that gives our lives meaning and make effort and practice and sacrifice worthwhile; and that we can figure out what that work is and how to rest to do it well. Further, I believe that the principle of deliberate rest can be adapted to any job and any workplace, whether you're a professional, a factory worker, a police officer, or a parent. If you recognize that work and rest are two sides of the same coin, that you can get more from rest by getting better at it and that by giving it a place in your life you'll stand a better chance of living the life you want, you'll be able to do your job, and your life's work, better.

The Problem of Rest

Only in recent history has "working hard" signaled
pride rather than shame.

—NASSIM NICHOLAS TALEB

IN HIS 1897 BOOK *Advice for a Young Investigator*, the
Spanish neuroscientist Santiago Ramón y Cajal warned
aspiring young scientists that two major impediments would
stand in their way as they tried to make new discoveries.
First, science had become a source of industrial and political
power, and growth of the scientific community, as well as
faster communication within the community through journals, conferences, and newspapers, had made science faster
and more competitive. No longer could scientists afford to
"concentrate for extended periods of time on one subject"
or think deeply "in the silence of the study, confident that
rivals would not disrupt their tranquil meditations." One
had to hurry to stay ahead of the competition. "Research is

now frantic," he warned, and this meant that fast, superficial science—and lots of it—won over slower, deeper, and more profound work.

Second, most scientists assumed that long hours were necessary to produce great work and that "an avalanche of lectures, articles, and books" would loosen some profound insight. This was one reason they willingly accepted a world of faster science: they believed it would make their own science better. But this was a style of work, Ramón y Cajal argued, that led to asking only shallow, easily answered questions rather than hard, fundamental ones. It created the appearance of profundity and feelings of productivity but did not lead to substantial discoveries. Choosing to be prolific, he contended, meant closing off the possibility of doing great work.

Although *Advice for a Young Investigator* was published in 1897, it is still worth reading. Ramón y Cajal was one of the founders of modern neuroscience: he helped prove that the nervous system was composed of many cells and developed staining techniques that made it possible to study neurons, the axons and dendrites along which signals pass between neurons, and the star-shaped glial cells that support the neurons. (The words *neuron, axon,* and *dendrite* were all coined between 1889 and 1896, when Ramón y Cajal, who was born in 1852, was himself a young investigator.) He was a deeply talented illustrator, and his drawings of the brain are still used by teachers. He published some three hundred articles and monographs during a career that lasted fifty years, on subjects ranging from neuroscience to public health to science fiction. When someone with his accomplishments offers advice, we should listen.

Ramón y Cajal's diagnosis of the challenges facing researchers remains timely. Complaints that modern life deprives us of opportunities for rest are as old as modern life itself, but even after more than a century, his argument that scientists are forced to trade quantity for quality, that overwork is the norm, and that the fast pace of scientific life discourages engagement and serious thinking, would resonate in any lecture hall today. And his recognition that this race to superficiality is driven by external and structural, as well as internal and cultural, forces is still a useful way to understand why we struggle to recognize the value of rest and make a place for it in our lives.

THE IDEA OF work and rest as opposites and competitors now seems perfectly logical, but it's one of those logical ideas that's actually a historical artifact. Before the eighteenth century, the boundaries between work and rest were not so clear-cut. Workplaces and domestic space were often intertwined: in the preindustrial era, skilled workers had shops in their homes, small farmers brought livestock into the house during winter months, scholars and teachers gave lessons out of their homes, and apprentices lived with their masters. Working time was more flexible and "task-oriented," as labor historian E. P. Thompson put it, and many workers sought to work only long enough to provide for their basic needs.

This order was upended by the Industrial Revolution in the eighteenth and nineteenth centuries. The factory and office came to be seen as the places where "real" work happened.

The home, in contrast, evolved into the domestic sphere, the place where a man could relax and recover from work. (Of course, men could believe that the home was a retreat from work so long as they did no work there; for women it was a different story.) The labor movement's advocacy of shorter hours, paid vacation days, and holidays further (though unintentionally) contributed to a sense that work and leisure were opposites and could be haggled over and won and lost.

The template of industrial labor, including its underlying assumptions about work and rest, was copied by service industries, professions, and bureaucracies in the mid-nineteenth century. The modern office was conceptualized as a machine for rationalizing and organizing intellectual labor, and it copied the working hours of factories. But the model has been an imperfect fit in creative industries, as it's extremely hard to measure productivity and quality in creative and knowledge work. In factories and fields, you can point to tangible products at the end of the day; in industries where the "product" is intangible and projects may take years to complete, it's harder to assess from day to day how you or your subordinates are performing.

But it is possible, especially in today's open office, to see who looks busy, who looks engaged, and who seems passionate about their work. As a result, service workers and professionals are rewarded not just for performing work but also for "performing" busyness at work. This has long been true, but with the growth of global twenty-four/seven enterprises and the proliferation of mobile and digital tools that let you work anywhere and anytime, let work follow you everywhere, and let employers track your activities in and out of the workplace, the opportunities for performing busyness expand. These tools give us the capacity to measure everything—except when to stop work, when to turn off our devices, and when to disconnect. Flexible hours often collapse into work hovering over all our hours, transforming work from something you break into smaller blocks and spread across the day into a flood that soaks your whole life. In the modern office, all the world's a stage, nowhere is off-camera, and the performance never stops.

Stories of consultants and law associates who schedule e-mail to go out in the middle of the night or workers who wear fatigue as a badge of honor update an old problem. In 1899 William James noted that that many Americans had gotten "into a wretched trick" of overwork and overextension, which increased "the frequency and severity of our breakdowns." An anonymous writer in Singapore's *Straits Times* observed in 1913, "The tendency of the present age is to mental overwork and the exhaustion of the brain force." Two years later, Bertie Charles Forbes noted that the modern industrialist "works harder than any of his workmen," and the banker "gets early to his office and performs more work—and brainier work—than any other three men in his nerve-wrecking profession." Such men had made America the envy of the world, he said, but they were "committing suicide by overwork."

Since the 1970s, a combination of forces has made the problem of overwork more pervasive. The service sectors in Western economies have grown dramatically while employment in manufacturing has declined. The erosion of labor unions and workplace protections has let employers push for longer hours while global competition, decreased job security, and flat wages (combined with rising housing prices in popular cities) have forced workers to work harder to stay in place. Corporations now shed staff in the course of restructuring and "process reengineering," forcing surviving workers to carry heavier workloads. Supporting tasks are outsourced to freelancers or contractors, who are struggling to adjust to an uncertain, feast-or-famine world. The 2008 recession and recovery has solidified a pattern in which companies seek to grow by increasing demands on existing workers rather than hiring new ones. A few industries have turned into fast-moving, winner-take-all contests: small numbers of people stand to make immense fortunes when their tech company goes public, their hedge fund investment pays off, or their song goes viral—and since no one knows how long they have until fashions change, technology evolves, or the bubble bursts, it makes sense to go all-in right now.

As a result, many of us actually are working longer hours. Working hours generally decline with increased productivity, but in the 1970s, increased productivity stopped yielding shorter working hours, despite the expectations of generations of economists. Working hours started to rise in the United States in the 1980s, especially among salaried workers and professionals like doctors, lawyers, bankers, and academics; in contrast, working hours (and full-time jobs and salaries) in less skilled, hourly professions began to fall. Since then, this split has spread to other parts of the world: today, well-off, well-educated people in Western Europe, Australia, and South Korea are also more likely to be overworked, while more poor people struggle to find stable jobs and face chronic underemployment. (Americans are still more likely to work nights and weekends, though, further cutting into their leisure time.)

We're not just spending more time at the office; informal work also absorbs more of our time. According to a 2015 Bureau of Labor Statistics report, in the United States parents of young children spend an average of seven hours every workday taking care of children. Earlier generations gave children more independence and mobility, but today's parenting is more time- and labor-intensive. This is one reason the amount of time spent on housework has barely budged in the last hundred years, despite the invention of dishwashers, washing machines, and other appliances.

We also spend more time commuting to work—and the proportion of people with long commutes is rising, too. In the UK, according to a 2015 study, roughly 3 million people, or 10 percent of the labor force, spent more than two hours a day commuting in 2014, a figure that had increased more than 70 percent since 2004. In the United States, workers spent an average of twenty-one minutes commuting in 1982; by 2014, that number had climbed to twenty-six minutes, with 17 percent of commuters spending forty-five minutes or more commuting. (The amount of time commuters spent stuck in traffic also rose, from sixteen hours a year in 1982 to forty-two hours a year in 2014.)

WE MAY SEE overwork and the marginalization of rest as a consequence of automation, globalization, the decline of unions, and the growth of a winner-take-all economy. But it also has an intellectual history, as Josef Pieper, a German Catholic theologian and professor of philosophical anthropology noted in a slender meditation on the place of leisure in modern society published just after World War II. *Muße und Kult* (or, as it was titled in the English translation, *Leisure: The Basis of Culture*) traced the history of Western thinking about how knowledge is produced, and how the rise of modern industry and bureaucracy changed how we think about intellectual activity. Indeed, Pieper would have noted that phrases like "producing knowledge" and "intellectual activity" are very modern: they assume that ideas are like manufactured goods and that knowledge workers (or symbolic analysts, as former secretary of labor Robert Reich calls them) are workers, presumptions that earlier eras would have found absurd. In ancient and medieval Europe, philosophers argued that the exercise of pure reason was never sufficient to make sense of the world. Knowledge (and the culture that formed through the accumulation of knowledge) required the marriage of logical and discursive methods (*ratio*) and contemplative practices and attitudes (*intellectus*). *Intellectus*, in turn, was enabled by leisure, which Pieper described as not just a "result of spare time" but "an attitude of non-activity, of inward calm." The philosopher's capacity for insight had its center in this "tranquil silence" that only the world's deep truths could disturb and that provided space for the cultivation of *intellectus*. Leisure was, as the English translation of *Muße und Kult* put it, the basis of culture.

Modern thinkers and industry destroyed this organic vision, Pieper argued. Immanuel Kant argued that only active intellectual effort could serve as a firm basis for knowledge; as he put it in 1796, "reason acquires its possessions through work," and forms of knowledge that claim anything other than formal, rational foundations are suspect. Cognition, Pieper wrote, became in the eighteenth century "an active, discursive labor of the *ratio*" alone, and *intellectus* and leisure were discarded.

Knowledge wasn't just the product of work; how hard you worked to produce it became a measure of how significant and profound the knowledge was. Disciplines that were hard to master, like physics and mathematics, came to be seen as more profound than softer (or easier) fields like botany and natural history, their knowledge closer to the realm of absolute and ultimate truth. Philosophy only mattered if it was the product of "herculean labor," as Kant put it. Anything created through contemplation (or religious revelation, or intuition) was, by definition, less impressive and trustworthy.

The rise of industry and technology, growth of the modern bureaucratic state, emergence of the modern office, rise of the labor movement, and triumph of the marketplace completed the transformation of knowledge from a product of leisure to a product of, well, production. The philosopher, writer, and scientist were all turned into "intellectual workers," their products subject to the regulation of the state and judgment of the marketplace. Some fought back. The nineteenth-century Romantic genius declared that he created only for himself and his muse and turned his back on the dictates of the market. Likewise, the liberal arts were reinvented as treasuries of timeless knowledge, a canon of great works stretching back to the beginnings of Western civilization. But these were small battles in a much larger war. By the mid-twentieth century, Pieper lamented, the conversion of thinkers into intellectual workers was complete: "The whole field of intellectual activity [has been] overwhelmed by the modern ideal of work and is at the mercy of its totalitarian claims," he wrote, while space for contemplation and leisure had been eliminated in the name of "planned diligence and 'total labor.'"

These philosophical arguments might seem arcane, but the assumptions that knowledge is produced rather than discovered or revealed, that the amount of work that goes into an idea determines its importance, and that the creation of ideas can be organized and institutionalized, all guide our thinking about work today. When we treat workaholics as heroes, we express a belief that labor rather than contemplation is the wellspring of great ideas and that the success of individuals and companies is a measure of their long hours. We take for granted that great companies are built by hard-driven, work-obsessed founders who inspire others to chase the next breakthrough and stay ahead of the competition. In a world where we're all encouraged to become entrepreneurs, figures like Steve Jobs and Elon Musk become the standards against which we're supposed to measure ourselves. It's not just executives who are workaholics: polymaths such as James

Franco, Dr. Dre, Madonna, Kanye West, and Gwen Stefani combine careers as actors, musicians, entrepreneurs, fashion designers, and authors. (People who make more money are also more likely to describe themselves as workaholics.)

Modern assumptions about knowledge as product and labor are also built into open office layouts meant to support collaboration between groups or spark serendipitous exchanges in the line at strategically placed water coolers. Such designs assume that new ideas emerge from a stochastic process of people and ideas bouncing off each other, from brainstorms and chance encounters, rather than from contemplation or deep thinking.

Santiago Ramón y Cajal argues that a view of science as demanding countless hours of dedicated effort—as a kind of "intellectual work," as Josef Pieper put it—leads investigators to waste their energy on small and superficial problems. However, he has a solution: the cultivation of "cerebral polarization or sustained concentration," a state of deep focus necessary to do great science.

The central feature of this state is a "steady orientation of all our faculties toward a single object of study for a period of months or even years." It is not enough to be smart, Ramón y Cajal warns: the "thinking of countless brilliant minds ends up sterile for lack of this ability." Just as an astronomer exposes a photographic plate for hours to "reveal stars so far away that even the most powerful telescopes fail to reveal them to the naked eye," so too are "time and concentration" needed to "allow the intellect to perceive a ray of light in the darkness of the most complex problem." Major discoveries require a "vigorous concentration of mental energy" to "raise to the conscious level" connections between observations made in the laboratory and "ideas slumbering in the unconscious."

This state of sustained concentration "refines judgment, enriches analytical powers, spurs constructive imagination, and—by focusing all light of reason on the darkness of a problem—allows unforeseen and subtle relationships to be discovered." Reaching it, he warns, requires "severe abstention and renunciation." One must avoid distractions like "malicious gossip" and newspapers, the "intellectual dispersion and waste of time required by social activity," and anything else that loosens "the creative tension of the mind" and "that quality of tone that nerve cells acquire when adapted to a particular subject." But this does not mean that the investigator should try to concentrate all the time. Diversions that are "light and promote the association of new ideas" are to be taken freely. Long walks, art, and music offer good material for a break. And if, after a period of sustained concentration, a breakthrough does not come, "yet we feel success is just around the corner, try resting for a while." A few weeks of "relaxation and quiet in the countryside brings calmness and clarity to the mind" and provides "intellectual refreshment." Even getting there can provide creative stimulus: "the powerful vibration of the locomotive and the spiritual solitude of the railway car," he says, will often "suggest ideas that are ultimately confirmed in the laboratory."

In other words, it is not constant effort that delivers results but a kind of constant, patient, unhurried focus that organizes the investigator's attention when at work and is present but watchful during periods of ease. Devoting yourself only to the first (to *ratio*, in other words) and neglecting the second (*intellectus*) might make you more productive in the short run but will make your work less profound in the long run.

The founder of neuroscience was onto something. His era lacked the tools to observe the brain as it functions, but if they had been available, Ramón y Cajal would have seen that when we rest and let our minds wander, our brains are almost as active as when we're concentrating hard on a problem. Further, while we're not conscious of it, the "resting" brain turns out to be consolidating memories, making sense of the past, and searching for solutions to problems that are occupying our waking hours.

The Science of Rest

The greatest geniuses sometimes accomplish more when they work less.

—ATTRIBUTED TO LEONARDO DA VINCI
IN GIORGIO VASARI'S *THE LIVES OF THE ARTISTS*

IN THE EARLY 1990s, Bharat Biswal, a graduate student at the Medical College of Wisconsin in Milwaukee, was trying to eliminate background noise in functional magnetic resonance imaging (fMRI) scans. fMRI provides a near-real-time view of the brain at work by measuring oxygen consumption in different parts of the brain. Just as you can tell who in a company is working late by seeing whose office lights are on, higher oxygen demand in an area of the brain means it's more active. fMRI was brand new at the time, and the effects it measures are incredibly small, so scientists were still figuring out how to filter the small, hard-to-read signals amid the background of ordinary brain activity and how to tell a real signal from random fluctuations or noise. Biswal had trained as an electrical engineer, but even after factoring out brain signals that regulate automatic functions like heart rate and breathing, he still couldn't get rid of a stubborn, low-frequency signal that the machines recorded when people were simply lying in them, doing nothing. Eventually, he concluded, it wasn't noise; it wasn't an artifact of the technology, or sampling technique, or signal-processing algorithm. Contrary to expectation, he was seeing a consistent pattern of activity in the brain's resting state. When he presented his findings at a local journal club, one senior colleague suggested that, as Biswal recalled, "I, along with my research, should be buried since this would destroy fMRI." Everyone knew that the resting brain didn't do anything interesting.

At about the same time that Biswal was being attacked in his journal club, Washington University School of Medicine professor Marcus Raichle was using positron emission tomography (PET) to map brain activity during reading. Cognitively, reading is a pretty complicated activity, since it can involve several different skills at once, from the recognition of letters to the interpretation of a phrase to the construction of a mental picture of a scene or comparison to a previous work, and neuroscientists are keen to understand how those connected regions (or *connectomes*) work together. In order to accurately measure how brain activity changes in response to external tasks, it's also important to have a baseline of comparison. Just as a doctor might want to know a patient's resting heart rate and blood pressure before measuring them during exercise, it's good to map a subject's brain when they're resting. When Raichle started looking at scans of people's brains when they weren't reading text but resting between tasks and staring at a blank screen, he was surprised to see that the subjects' brains didn't just quiet down; instead, a second, different set of regions switched on. When people turned their attention outward again, that region switched off, and other regions lit up. This resting-state activity wasn't just scattered or random, either; it was as coordinated as when people were reading.

These studies convinced Biswal, Raichle, and other neuroscientists that the resting brain isn't inactive. The brain automatically switches on a default mode network (DMN), a series of interconnected sections that activate as soon as people stop concentrating on external tasks, and shifts from outward-focused to inward-focused cognition. As they've explored it further, scientists have realized that the DMN and resting state are doing critical work on our behalf. They've found that the DMNs of people who score high on creativity tests differ from those of people who are average: some regions of their resting brains are more active and there are higher levels of connectivity between some regions, while other regions are less tightly integrated. Further, in these people, some of the same areas that are active when they're concentrating on work are still switched on when they just stare into space; even when they've stopped trying to think about problems, their brains still plug away, generating ideas that they'll use when they return to work. This research has revolutionized our understanding of what happens when we rest.

ONE STRIKING CHARACTERISTIC of the brain in its resting state is that it's barely less energetic than the engaged brain. Even when you're staring into space, your brain consumes only slightly less energy than it does when you're solving differential equations. We can drop into the resting state literally in the blink of an eye: the DMN can switch on and off in the fraction of a second it takes to blink. So why does the brain seem to want to return to the resting state?

As they've have mapped and compared the brains of different people, scientists have discovered that there are variations in the structures of DMNs. Some of these variations are age-related: DMNs change as we move from childhood into adolescence and adulthood. Some variations correlate to different cognitive strengths. To some degree these may be natural, but they're also the product of training, in much the same way the bodies of swimmers, football players, and gymnasts differ.

Some people's resting brains show greater levels of communication between different regions, or what neuroscientists call resting-state functional connectivity. These stronger connections predict enhanced cognitive abilities, like better performance on fluid intelligence tests and language ability. They can also correlate to achievements and outlook: various resting-state functional connectivity patterns can predict educational level and income, levels of life satisfaction, executive control, and focus. Other scientists have found that the complexity of the DMN shapes our capacity for self-awareness, memory, ability to imagine the future, empathy, and moral judgment.

The connection between development of the DMN and psychological development in children is especially striking. Mary Helen Immordino-Yang, an expert in child psychology, education, and neuroscience at the University of Southern California, and her colleagues have found that children whose brains demonstrate greater levels of connectivity in the resting state tend to have superior reading skills, better memory, and higher scores on intelligence and attention tests. It also relates to their levels of empathy and ability to imagine playmates' and parents' points of view: the better-developed your DMN, other scientists have found, the better able you are to construct models of other people's minds.

There are also correlations between a damaged DMN and cognitive impairment or mental illness. Children with less-well-developed DMNs or delayed maturation of their DMNs are more likely to exhibit psychopathologies. The DMN is more active and harder to control in people suffering from depression. The brains of people with post-traumatic stress disorder, obsessive-compulsive disorder, and memory loss have DMNs that are structured and act differently than those in healthy brains: some subsystems that are connected in healthy brains are decoupled, while other subsystems are working more frantically. People who suffer from attention deficits after traumatic brain injury have reduced connectivity in their default mode network. Patients with depression or schizophrenia and people on the autism spectrum have DMNs that are more active and harder to control. (Indeed, hyperconnectivity may be a strategy the brain uses to respond to injury.) Amyloid beta, the protein that triggers the buildup of amyloid plaque in the brain and the onset of Alzheimer's disease, seems to do special damage to the default network.

In other words, a set of activities that we're not conscious of (pretty much by definition), and which we didn't even know existed until the 1990s, turns out to be implicated in just about every significant cognitive and emotional activity. Intelligence? Check. Moral and emotional judgment? Check. Empathy? Yep. Sanity? Check.

That's a lot of benefit for something we call "rest." And if your "resting" brain is much more active than you realize, giving your brain the right kinds of "rest" is critical to its development, health, and productivity.

WHILE RAICHLE AND other neuroscientists were using PET and fMRI to map the brain's default mode network and explore connections between the structure of those networks and cognitive and emotional abilities, another group of scientists were starting to study a different but equally elusive phenomenon: task-unrelated thinking, or, as it's more commonly called, mind-wandering. Task-unrelated thinking is inward-focused and unconnected to external activity. Your mind naturally wanders when you're doing something that's automatic or involves muscle memory, like folding clothes or knitting or driving on a familiar road. Mind-wandering can take a pleasant form, like a reverie or mental replay of some happy event, or it may involve brooding over something bad. For a long time, the conventional wisdom was that mind-wandering was always negative. In everyday usage, the term *mind-wandering* is synonymous with distraction and lost time. For some, it's a source of embarrassment: the most vivid memories of mind-wandering may be when a teacher calls on you when you're staring out the window or a coach yells at you to "get your head in the game." Most of the time we can't recall what we were thinking about as our minds wandered, which makes it hard to believe that anything productive comes from mind-wandering.

But some psychologists argue that mind-wandering is more than a mental lapse. For one thing, as psychologist Jonathan Smallwood notes, a lot of sophisticated cognitive activity is undirected: without having to tell ourselves to do so, we can recognize faces, recall memories, read emotions, and remember old songs. Cognition often "organizes itself on behalf of the person," Smallwood says, without our conscious direction. Further, Smallwood says, our minds seem to be "designed to engage in cognition that isn't confined by the environment." People spend a lot of time engaged in unconscious or inward-focused thought: by some estimates, up to half our waking hours are spent mind-wandering. Something that we do that much of, and we do so easily, ought to have some benefit.

Just like the default mode network, mind-wandering turns out to be implicated in a number of important mental processes. Michael Corballis, a psychologist and expert on memory and mind-wandering, notes that during mind-wandering our minds often head toward the past or future. We remember episodes from our childhood, daydream about what life would be like if we got that big promotion, or simply imagine what we might make for dinner. These activities often have more of a purpose than we recognize. Sifting through memories can let us imagine another person's perspective on events or think about what we could have done differently. Imagining future events can help us prepare for them. And often, we comb through the past to prepare for the future: we replay the past to make sense of our history, not to preserve the accuracy of our memories.

There's a third major place the mind goes when it wanders: to problems we've been working on. But compared to its conscious, directed state, the wandering mind deals with problems in a looser, freer way. In fact, it looks to Corballis like "mind-wandering is the secret of creativity."

In their effort to measure creativity in the lab, scientists often use simple tests to measure two kinds of thinking: convergent thinking and divergent thinking. Convergent thinking requires seeing connections between apparently different things; divergent thinking requires finding new uses for or meanings in familiar things. A classic convergence-thinking test is the Remote Associates Test (RAT), in which you have to find the common association between three apparently unrelated words. (For example, what do *fly*, *stool*, and *none* share? Adding the word *bar* in front of them creates a common word or phrase. What word connects *playing*, *credit*, and *yellow*? The answer is *card*.) Convergent thinking requires cleverness and speed, but it isn't considered that creative; it's more like solving a puzzle than proving a theorem. Divergent thinking, in contrast, is more creative and open-ended. It's commonly tested by asking subjects to come up with many novel uses of a common item, like a spool of thread, or a spoon, or a chair, and then grading their results on the basis of originality, fluency, flexibility, and elaboration.

As psychologist Benjamin Baird and his colleagues discovered, a little mind-wandering during focused tasks can boost creative thinking. Baird administrated the Alternative Uses Test (a divergent-thinking test where you have to come up with novel uses for an ordinary item, like a straw or a chair) to 145 students. They then assigned each student to one of four groups. The first group immediately did another AUT. The other three had several minutes to incubate ideas; during those minutes, one group sat quietly, another had to do a demanding task, the third an undemanding task. When Baird compared the scores of the first and second rounds, the group that did a second AUT immediately did worse the second time, as you might expect. The members of the demanding task group improved slightly, while the resting group actually dropped a bit. The jokers in the pack were the undemanding task group: they were 40 percent more creative the second time and outperformed everybody else by a wide margin. Having to do the simple task didn't wreck their creativity; on the contrary, because it gave them the chance to do a little mind-wandering, members of the fourth group had time to subconsciously work on the AUT.

An experiment conducted by Ap Dijksterhuis and his colleagues at the University of Amsterdam likewise found that brief periods of mind-wandering boost creativity. In their experiment, students had four minutes to evaluate four different car models. The task required them to weigh a number of different features and select the best vehicle. Students who also did a simple anagram puzzle during those four minutes consistently made better choices than those who were left undisturbed.

Researchers have also found that a small amount of background noise can boost creativity and that some people perform better on creativity tests when listening to music. This is why some people like working in cafés: the low buzz of conversations and comings and goings provides a useful stimulus, loosening the mind just enough to encourage associative thinking but not so much as to really drive you off task.

Experiments show that when people are engaged in creative tasks, their brains draw on areas that are also prominent in the DMN. In one study, when people were placed in an fMRI machine and had to make up creative stories based on sets of words that flashed on a screen, their brains drew more heavily on two areas active in the DMN, the bilateral medial frontal gyri and left anterior cingulate cortex; in contrast, when they were told to make up dull stories, these regions stayed relatively quiet. In another study, thirty people took a version of the Alternative Uses Test while in an fMRI machine. When people gave more original answers, their brains showed higher levels of activation in the ventral anterior cingulate cortex, another area that is active when the DMN switches on. Mind-wandering, it seems, enhances creativity by tapping into the DMN and its ability to reach across and connect regions of the brain that don't normally work together during directed cognition.

Other studies have revealed that the brains of creative people display stronger-than-normal connections between certain areas within the DMN or greater connectivity between the DMN and others regions associated with particular skills. A comparison of high-achieving and low-achieving professors at a Chinese university found that the brains of more eminent academics had more regional grey matter volume in the left inferior frontal gyrus and greater levels of connectivity within the creative sections of the DMN. Tohoku University's Hikaru Takeuchi, a researcher on aging, and colleagues found a correlation between levels of functional connectivity in the DMN and performance on divergent-thinking tests. A study by scientists at Southwest University in Chongqing found that the resting-state brains of students who scored higher on the Torrance Tests of Creative Thinking, which measure how creative someone is, showed stronger connections between the medial prefrontal cortex and the middle temporal gyrus regions within the DMN. Scientists at the University of Graz who compared the resting brains of a group of people who scored high on divergent-thinking tests to those of a low-scoring group found that the more creative group showed greater levels of connectivity between the DMN and another region of the brain, the inferior prefrontal cortex.

Just as great athletes seem able to draw on reserves of energy that the rest of us cannot or are more effective at getting oxygen to tired brains and muscles, so too do the DMNs of creative people have stronger connections between areas associated with functional abilities like verbal acuity, visual skill, and memory, connections that allow their brains to keep working on problems when in the resting state.

There also appear to be a few areas of the DMN that are less active or tightly integrated in creative people. According to one model of creative thinking, new ideas are created in a two-step process: first, the brain generates lots of ideas, and second, it evaluates them. Ideas that are both novel and original are passed on from the unconscious to the conscious mind. The generative and evaluative functions are thought to take place in different parts of the brain, both of which are part of the DMN. In this theory one would expect that in creative people, the generative function would have more freedom to produce ideas, and the evaluative function would be less tightly integrated into the DMN.

And, in fact, University of Haifa neuroscientist Naama Mayseless has found an association between creative ability and lowered activity in the evaluative center of the brain. She gave thirty people the Torrance Test, and then they took a second test in an fMRI machine in which they were given the names of objects and their uses and asked to evaluate whether or not the use was original. For example, if the object was "surfboard" and the use was "picnic table," most people would call that an original use. What Mayseless wanted to observe was what happened in people's brains during the evaluation process, which areas were more or less active, and how that activity correlated to performance on the Torrance Test. She found that subjects who had scored higher on the Torrance Test demonstrated lower activity in the left temporoparietal and inferior frontal regions, suggesting that these areas of the brain are associated with evaluation of originality, and that those regions—and thus the evaluative function—are less active in creative people.

Studies of paradoxical functional facilitation, in which people who've had brain injuries, strokes, or degenerative brain diseases affecting the left temporoparietal region—the part of the brain where the evaluative center resides—suddenly develop new creative abilities or an obsession with painting or playing music, also provide evidence for the two-stage model of creative cognition. In one especially compelling case, a forty-six-year-old Israeli accountant developed an interest in drawing days after having a stroke. He had never studied art, but he was sketching and then painting while in the hospital; at home a month later, he was turning out several works a day. As his recovery proceeded and his old cognitive abilities returned, though, his artistic abilities receded; after eight months, he was back to normal, and he could no longer paint. A series of MRI scans taken immediately after the stroke and during his recovery showed what was happening as his brief artistic career waxed and waned: a hemorrhagic stroke had flooded the left side of his brain with blood, suppressing the evaluative function in the left temporoparietal region; as the blood drained and the region recovered, his brain's evaluative function improved and his artistic ability declined.

Together, these studies suggest that the default mode network is a source of raw creative energy, that the default networks of creative people are organized differently than those of normal people, and that more creative people are better able to tap that energy. This is not to say that these studies provide a definitive view of how the creative brain works. We know more about the workings of the human brain than ever, but we're still a long way from being able to answer really big questions about how creativity works and how to make it work better. Electroencephalography (EEG), which detects electrical activity in the brain, works in near real-time, but it has low spatial resolution; further, since scientists are trying to detect changes of a few microvolts against a background of fifty to two hundred microvolts of normal brain activity, they have to run the same tests hundreds to times to find statistically meaningful changes. PET and fMRI require subjects to lie still, so we can't use them to study the brains of painters or craftspeople, or people who think on their feet. fMRI doesn't record brain activity by tracking firing neurons; it shows which parts of the brain are active by identifying tiny changes in blood flow and oxygen consumption. The data analysis methods scientists use to probe connections between brain activity and cognitive activity are still primitive. When a pair of neuroscientists tried to apply those methods to understand how a simple computer chip works, for example, they found that they could "not meaningfully describe the hierarchy of information processing in the processor"; as they diplomatically put it, "current approaches in neuroscience may fall short of producing meaningful models of the brain." Finally, psychologists argue over how good a job divergence tests do of measuring creativity, and how much the "small c" creativity used in solving problems on tests or in everyday life resembles the "big C" of artistic and scientific creativity. Neuroscience is nothing short of remarkable, but we should recognize its limits even as we admire its accomplishments.

STUDIES OF THE default mode network and mind-wandering help us make sense of a phenomenon that has long puzzled psychologists. Many famous stories of problem-solving or creative breakthroughs begin with a period of intense work and focus, during which the scientist or artist or writer pores over evidence, labors over theories, and struggles toward an answer. Frustrated and tired, she stops for a break and turns her attention to something else. Days or weeks later, a solution suddenly appears; she hadn't been thinking about the problem, but in a flash, the answer is suddenly present in her mind, as clear as day. She then returns to the problem and verifies that the insight is correct.

This is a model described by English psychologist Graham Wallas in his 1926 book *The Art of Thought*. After studying accounts of creative breakthroughs and moments of insight, Wallas concluded that they follow a four-stage process. The first stage, preparation, consists of all the visible, conscious activity necessary in modern creative and productive work. It's where you formulate a problem, read, sketch, write, tinker, and think. You apply formal methods, ponder the details, and try to work your way to a solution. It's easy to disparage this labor, but most creative breakthroughs happen when you're immersed in a problem, familiar with all its parts, and examining it from every angle. Just as a great musician can play an instrument without thinking about it, so too must you be so fluent with ideas and arguments that your subconscious can play with them. So the preparation phase is absolutely necessary in creative thinking. Sometimes that works, but with big problems, often you hit a wall.

To get past a mental block, whether you're working with brainteasers or brain science, you have to move on to the next stage in Wallas's model: incubation. With small problems, such as crossword puzzles or riddles, the incubation phase may only last seconds or minutes. For much bigger problems, incubation might stretch out for weeks or months.

At some point, though, the answer will feel within reach. At this point, Wallas warns, it is important not to force it, as returning your attention to the problem "may have the effect of interrupting or hindering it." Instead, you have to trust that your unconscious will drive to the third phase, illumination, the moment when the answer bursts into your consciousness. These a-ha moments are famous and memorable precisely because they're so striking. They feel like they "occur suddenly, without exertion, like an inspiration," as German physicist Hermann von Helmholtz said. From there, it is on to the verification phase: you set the solution on a logical foundation, fill in the details, or fit it into a bigger project. Like preparation, verification is largely a conscious, formal activity. It's something you can train yourself or others to do and something you can make more efficient, just like any job. You can't say the same thing about incubation or illumination.

Or can you? Despite their elusive and evasive properties, might it be possible that we can treat incubation and illumination as skills and discover ways to make them more dependable? When *The Art of Thought* was published, psychologists had no tools for measuring brain activity: German psychiatrist Hans Berger was still developing EEG and would not announce his invention and the first measurements of brain waves until 1929. The discovery of the brain's default mode network and the importance of mind-wandering, however, lets us fill in the gaps in Wallas's work. We now know that our resting brains and wandering minds are actually quite active. We know that the areas recruited during spontaneous cognition aren't hard-wired and fixed but evolve and grow and strengthen over time. We know that the structure of default mode and creative networks can change over time, through training or trauma or aging. And we're beginning to see how we can tap into and improve the resting brain's ability to help us generate insights, see novel connections, and make breakthroughs.

I'm not talking about experimenting with nootropic drugs or do-it-yourself electrical brain stimulation (though there are people who advocate both). Whether they know it or not, creative people treat incubation and illumination like skills every day. That's why they develop and refine daily routines and practices that preserve time for mind-wandering, sharpen their sensitivity to insights, and allow them to capture moments of illumination. That's why they spend their lives feeding their curiosity and nurturing their instincts, trusting, as Finnish neuroscientist Ragnar Granit put it in 1972, that they would "very gradually build up living and creative structures" that would support great insights. (Even though he was a Nobel Prize–winner, Granit confessed, "We do not know how the brain" builds its unconscious ability. "We simply have to admit that the brain is designed that way.") Henri Poincaré, who said that illumination rarely happens "except after some days of voluntary effort which has appeared absolutely fruitless and whence nothing good seems to have come," had great respect for the cultivated unconscious. It was, he thought, "in no way inferior to" his conscious mind; in fact, it "knows better how to divine [answers] than the conscious self, since it succeeds where that has failed."

Graham Wallas did have a suggestion for those who wanted to better understand incubation and illumination. He noted that "in the case of the more difficult forms of creative thought," it was important that during incubation "nothing should interfere with the free working of the unconscious or partial conscious processes of the mind. In those cases, the stage of Incubation should include a large amount of actual mental relaxation. It would, indeed, be interesting to examine, from that point of view, the biographies of a couple hundred original thinkers and writers."

Such an undertaking, he hoped, could yield some insights into how rest stimulates creativity; it might even inspire "the formulation of a few rules." The discovery of the creative potential of the resting brain gives us a foundation on which to build a biographical structure. Let's see what an examination of creative lives reveals, and what it can teach us.

PART I

Stimulating Creativity

We must take advantage of all lucid moments, whether they occur during the meditation following prolonged rest; during the super-intense mental work nerve cells achieve when fired by concentration; or during scientific discussion, whose impact often generates unanticipated intuition like sparks from steel.

—SANTIAGO RAMÓN Y CAJAL,
ADVICE FOR A YOUNG INVESTIGATOR

Four Hours

Four or five hours daily—it is not much to ask; but one day must tell another, one week certify another, one month bear witness to another of the same story, and you will acquire a habit by which the one-talent man will earn a high interest, and by which the ten-talent man may at least save his capital.

—WILLIAM OSLER

WHEN YOU EXAMINE the lives of history's most creative figures, you are immediately confronted with a paradox: they organize their lives around their work, but not their days.

Figures as different as Charles Dickens, Henri Poincaré, and Ingmar Bergman, working in disparate fields in different times, all shared a passion for their work, a terrific ambition to succeed, and an almost superhuman capacity to focus. Yet when you look closely at their daily lives, they only spent a few hours a day doing what we would recognize as their most important work. The rest of the time, they were hiking mountains, taking naps, going on walks with friends, or just sitting and thinking. Their creativity and productivity, in other words, were not the result of endless hours of toil. Their towering creative achievements result from modest "working" hours.

How did they manage to be so accomplished? Can a generation raised to believe that eighty-hour workweeks are necessary for success learn something from the lives of the people who directed *Wild Strawberries*, laid the foundations of chaos theory and topology, and wrote *Great Expectations*?

I think we can. If some of history's greatest figures didn't put in immensely long hours, maybe the key to unlocking the secret of their creativity lies in understanding not just how they labored but how they rested, and how the two relate.

Let's start by looking at the lives of two figures. They were both very accomplished in their fields. Conveniently, they were next-door neighbors and friends who lived in the village of Downe, southeast of London. And, in different ways, their lives offer an entrée into the question of how labor, rest, and creativity connect.

First, imagine a silent, cloaked figure walking home on a dirt path winding through the countryside. On some mornings he walks with his head down, apparently lost in thought. On others he walks slowly and stops to listen to the woods around him, a habit "which he practiced in the tropical forests of Brazil" during his service as a naturalist in the Royal Navy, collecting animals, studying the geography and geology of South America, and laying the foundations for a career that would reach its peak with the publication of *The Origin of Species* in 1859. Now, Charles Darwin is older and has turned from collecting to theorizing. Darwin's ability to move silently reflects his own concentration and need for quiet. Indeed, his son Francis said, Darwin could move so stealthily he once came upon "a vixen playing with her cubs at only a few feet distance" and often greeted foxes coming home from their nocturnal hunts.

Had those same foxes crossed paths with Darwin's next-door neighbor, the baronet John Lubbock, they would have run for their lives. Lubbock liked to start the day with a ride through the country with his hunting dogs. If Darwin was a bit like Mr. Bennet in *Pride and Prejudice*, a respectable gentleman of moderate means who was polite and conscientious but preferred the company of family and books, Lubbock was more like Mr. Bingley, extroverted and enthusiastic, and wealthy enough to move easily in society and life. As he aged, Darwin was plagued by various ailments; even in his sixties, Lubbock still had "the lounging grace of manner which is peculiar to the Sixth-Form Eton boy," according to one visitor. But the neighbors shared a love of science, even though their working lives were as different as their personalities.

After his morning walk and breakfast, Darwin was in his study by eight and worked a steady hour and a half. At nine thirty he would read the morning mail and write letters. Downe was far away enough from London to discourage casual visitors, yet close enough to allow the morning mail to reach correspondents and colleagues in the city in just a few hours. At ten thirty, Darwin returned to more serious work, sometimes moving to his aviary, greenhouse, or one of several other buildings where he conducted his experiments. By noon, he would declare, "I've done a good day's work," and set out on a long walk on the Sandwalk, a path he had laid out not long after buying Down House. (Part of the Sandwalk ran through land leased to Darwin by the Lubbock family.) When he returned after an hour or more, Darwin had lunch and answered more letters. At three he would retire for a nap; an hour later he would arise, take another walk around the Sandwalk, then return to his study until five thirty, when he would join his wife, Emma, and their family for dinner. On this schedule he wrote nineteen books, including technical volumes on climbing plants, barnacles, and other subjects; the controversial *Descent of Man*; and *The Origin of Species*, probably the single most famous book in the history of science, and a book that still affects the way we think about nature and ourselves.

Anyone who reviews his schedule cannot help but notice the creator's paradox. Darwin's life revolved around science. Since his undergraduate days, Darwin had devoted himself to scientific collecting, exploration, and eventually theorizing. He and Emma moved to the country from London to have more space to raise a family and to have more space— in more than one sense of the word—for science. Down House gave him space for laboratories and greenhouses, and the countryside gave him the peace and quiet necessary to work. But at the same time, his days don't seem very busy to us. The times we would classify as "work" consist of three ninety-minute periods. If he had been a professor in a university today, he would have been denied tenure. If he'd been working in a company, he would have been fired within a week.

It's not that Darwin was careless about his time or lacked ambition. Darwin was intensely time-conscious and, despite being a gentleman of means, felt that he had none to waste. While sailing around the world on the HMS *Beagle*, he wrote to his sister Susan Elizabeth that "a man who dares to waste one hour of time has not discovered the value of life." When he was deciding whether or not to marry, one of his concerns was that "loss of time—cannot read in the evenings," and in his journals he kept an account of the time he lost to chronic illness. His "pure love" of science was "much aided by the ambition to be esteemed by my fellow naturalists," he confessed in his autobiography. He was passionate and driven, so much so that he was given to anxiety attacks over his ideas and their implications.

John Lubbock is far less well-known than Darwin, but at the time of his death in 1913 he was "one of the most accomplished of England's amateur men of science, one of the most prolific and successful authors of his time, one of the most earnest of social reformers, and one of the most successful law-makers in the recent history of Parliament." Lubbock's scientific interests ranged across paleontology, animal psychology, and entomology—he invented the ant farm—but his most enduring work was in archaeology. His writings popularized the terms *Paleolithic* and *Neolithic*, which archaeologists still use today. His purchase of Avebury, an ancient settlement southwest of London, saved its stone monuments from destruction by developers. Today, it rivals Stonehenge in popularity and archaeological importance, and its preservation earned him the title Baron Avebury in 1900.

Lubbock's accomplishments were not just in science. He inherited his father's prosperous bank and turned it into a power in late Victorian finance. He helped modernize the British banking system. He spent decades in Parliament, where he was a successful and well-regarded legislator. His biography lists twenty-nine books, a number of them best sellers that were translated into many foreign languages. Lubbock's output was prodigious, notable even to his high-achieving contemporaries. "How you find time" for science, writing, politics, and business "is a mystery to me," Charles Darwin told him in 1881.

It might be tempting to imagine Lubbock as a modern equivalent of today's hard-charging alpha male, a kind of steampunk Tony Stark. Yet here's a twist: his fame as a politician rested on an advocacy of rest. Britain's bank holidays—four national holidays for everyone—were his invention, and they sealed his popular reputation when they went into effect in 1871. So beloved were they, and so closely associated with him, the popular press christened them "St. Lubbock's Days." He spent decades championing the Early Closing Bill, which limited working hours for people under eighteen to seventy-four hours (!) per week; when the legislation finally passed in April 1903, thirty years after he first took up the cause, it was referred to as "Avebury's Bill."

This public advocacy of rest wasn't an effort to play to the mob. The baron and banker was no calculating populist. Lubbock seems to have been genuinely sympathetic to the plight of workers, but he was still unapologetically aristocratic. He played with other future dukes and earls at an elementary school that his biographer called a "House of youthful Lords"; it was almost a step down the social ladder to go on to Eton. At his home, High Elms, and on his extensive travels he spent time in the company of presidents, prime ministers, royalty, leading scientists, and artists.

And Lubbock practiced what he preached. It could be hard to manage his time when Parliament was in session, as debates and votes could extend well after midnight, but at High Elms he was up at six thirty, and after prayers, a ride, and breakfast, he started work at eight thirty. He divided his day into half-hour blocks, a habit he'd learned from his father. After long years of practice, he was able to switch his attention from "some intricate point of finance" with his partners or clients to "such a problem in biology as parthenogenesis" without skipping a beat. In the afternoons he would spend a couple more hours outdoors. He was an enthusiastic cricketer, "a fast, left under-hand bowler" who regularly brought professional players to High Elms to coach him. His younger brothers played football; two of them played in the very first FA Cup finals in 1872. He was also fond of fives, a handball-like sport that he mastered at Eton. Later in life, when he took up golf, Lubbock replaced the cricket pitch at High Elms with a nine-hole course.

So despite their differences in personality and the different quality of their achievements, both Darwin and Lubbock managed something that seems increasingly alien today. Their lives were full and memorable, their work was prodigious, and yet their days are also filled with downtime.

This looks like a contradiction, or a balance that's beyond the reach of most of us. It's not. As we will see, Darwin and Lubbock, and many other creative and productive figures, weren't accomplished despite their leisure; they were accomplished because of it. And even in today's twenty-four/seven, always-on world, we can learn how to blend work and rest together in ways that make us smarter, more creative, and happier.

DARWIN IS NOT the only famous scientist who combined a lifelong dedication to science with apparently short working hours. We can see similar patterns in many others' careers, and it's worth starting with the lives of scientists for several reasons. Science is a competitive, all-consuming enterprise. Scientists' accomplishments—the number of articles and books they write, the awards they win, the rate at which their works are cited—are well-documented and easy to measure and compare. As a result, their legacies are often easier to determine than those of business leaders or famous figures. At the same time, scientific disciplines are quite different from each other, which gives us a useful variety in working habits and personalities. Additionally, most scientists have not been subjected to the kind of intense mythmaking that surrounds, and alternately magnifies and obscures, business leaders and politicians. We may have to sort out rumor from truth when studying scientists, but rarely are we confronted with an active force field of PR and spin.

Finally, a number of scientists were themselves interested in the ways work and rest affect thinking and contribute to inspiration. One example is Henri Poincaré, the French mathematician whose public eminence and accomplishments placed him on a level similar to Darwin. Poincaré's thirty books and five hundred papers spanned number theory, topology, astronomy and celestial mechanics, theoretical and applied physics, and philosophy; the American mathematician Eric Temple Bell described him as "the last universalist." He was involved in efforts to standardize time zones, supervised railway development in northern France (he was educated as a mining engineer), served as inspector general of the Corps des Mines, and was a professor at the Sorbonne.

Poincaré wasn't just famous among his fellow scientists: in 1895 he was, along with the novelist Émile Zola, sculptors Auguste Rodin and Jules Dalou, and composer Camille Saint-Saëns, the subject of a study by French psychiatrist Édouard Toulouse on the psychology of genius. Toulouse noted that Poincaré kept very regular hours. He did his hardest thinking between 10 a.m. and noon, and again between five and seven in the afternoon. The nineteenth century's most towering mathematical genius worked just enough to get his mind around a problem—about four hours a day.

We see the same pattern among other noted mathematicians. G. H. Hardy, one of Britain's leading mathematicians in the first half of the twentieth century, would start his day with a leisurely breakfast and close reading of the cricket scores, then from nine to one would be immersed in mathematics. After lunch he would be out again, walking and playing tennis. "Four hours creative work a day is about the limit for a mathematician," he told his friend and fellow Oxford professor C. P. Snow. Hardy's longtime collaborator John Edensor Littlewood believed that the "close concentration" required to do serious work meant that a mathematician could work "four hours a day or at most five, with breaks about every hour (for walks perhaps)." Littlewood was famous for always taking Sundays off, claiming that it guaranteed he would have new ideas when he returned to work on Monday. Even in the early 1900s, this was unusual: Littlewood later recalled that "my generation worked mainly at night, and 1 o'clock was early to go to bed: there was also a monstrous belief that 8 hours was the minimum a mathematician should work a day." The Hungarian American mathematician Paul Halmos likewise confessed, "I seemed to have psychic energy for only three or four hours of work, 'real work,' each day"; yet that gave him enough time to make fundamental contributions to half a dozen specialties.

A survey of scientists' working lives conducted in the early 1950s yielded results in a similar range. Illinois Institute of Technology psychology professors Raymond Van Zelst and Willard Kerr surveyed their colleagues about their work habits and schedules, then graphed the number of hours faculty spent in the office against the number of articles they produced.

You might expect that the result would be a straight line showing that the more hours scientists worked, the more articles they published. But it wasn't. The data revealed an M-shaped curve. The curve rose steeply at first and peaked at between ten to twenty hours per week. The curve then turned downward. Scientists who spent twenty-five hours in the workplace were no more productive than those who spent five. Scientists working thirty-five hours a week were half as productive as their twenty-hours-a-week colleagues.

From there, the curve rose again, but more modestly. Researchers who buckled down and spent fifty hours per week in the lab were able to pull themselves out of the thirty-five-hour valley: they became as productive as colleagues who spent five hours a week in the lab. Van Zelst and Kerr speculated that this fifty-hour bump was concentrated in "physical research which requires continuous use of bulky equipment," and that most of those ten-hour days were spent tending machines and occasionally taking measurements.

After that, it was all downhill: the sixty-plus-hour-a-week researchers were the least productive of all.

Van Zelst and Kerr also asked faculty how many "hours per typical work day do you devote to home work which contributes to the efficient performance of your job" and graphed those results against productivity as well. This time, they didn't see an M but rather a single curve peaking around three to three and a half hours a day. Unfortunately, they don't say anything about total hours spent working at the office and home; they only allude to "the probability that" the most productive researchers "do much of their creative work at home or elsewhere," rather than on campus. If you assume that the most productive office and home workers in this study are the same, this cohort is working between twenty-five and thirty-eight hours a week. In a six-day week, that works out to an average of four to six hours a day.

You see a similar convergence of four- to five-hour-long working days in the lives of writers. The German writer and Nobel laureate Thomas Mann had settled into a daily work schedule by 1910, when he was thirty-five and had published the acclaimed novel *Buddenbrooks*. Mann started the day at nine, shutting himself in his office with strict instructions not to be disturbed and working first on novels. After lunch, the "afternoons are for reading, for my much too mountainous correspondence and for walks," he said. After an hour-long nap and afternoon tea, he would spend another hour or two working on easy short pieces and editing.

Anthony Trollope, the great nineteenth-century English novelist, likewise kept a strict writing schedule. In an account of his life at Waltham House, where he lived from 1859 to 1871, he described his mature working style. At five o'clock in the morning, a servant arrived with coffee. He first read over the previous day's work, then at five thirty set his watch on his desk and started writing. He wrote a thousand words an hour, an average of forty finished pages a week, until it was time to leave for his day job at the post office at eight o'clock. Working this way, he published forty-seven novels before his death in 1882 at the age of sixty-seven, though he gave little indication that he regarded this as remarkable, perhaps because his mother, who started writing in her fifties to support her family, published more than a hundred books. He wrote, "All those I think who have lived as literary men,—working daily as literary labourers—will agree with me that three hours a day will produce as much as a man ought to write."

Trollope's steady working hours were matched by his contemporary Charles Dickens. After an early life burning the midnight oil, Dickens settled into a schedule as "methodical or orderly" as a "city clerk," his son Charley said. Dickens shut himself in his study from nine until two, with a break for lunch. Most of his novels were serialized in magazines, and Dickens was rarely more than a chapter or two ahead of the illustrators and printer. Nonetheless, after five hours, Dickens was done for the day.

While this kind of discipline might seem to be an expression of Victorian strictness, many prolific twentieth-century authors worked this way, too. Like Trollope, Egyptian novelist Naguib Mahfouz worked as a civil servant, and he mainly wrote fiction in the late afternoon, from 4:00 p.m. to 7:00 p.m. Canadian writer Alice Munro, who won the 2013 Nobel Prize in Literature, wrote from 8:00 a.m. to 11:00 a.m. Australian novelist Peter Carey said, "I think three hours is fine" for a day's work; such a schedule allowed him to write thirteen novels, including two Booker Prize winners. Norman Maclean, author of *A River Runs Through It*, wrote every morning from nine to noon; so did Swedish director Ingmar Bergman and the Icelandic novelist and Nobel laureate Halldór Laxness. W. Somerset Maugham worked "only four hours" a day, until 1:00 p.m.—"but never less," he added.

Gabriel García Márquez wrote each day for five hours. Ernest Hemingway would start work about six in the morning and finish before noon. Unless deadlines were looming, Saul Bellow would retreat to his study after breakfast, write until lunch, and then review his day's work. Irish novelist Edna O'Brien would work in the morning, "stop around one or two and spend the rest of the afternoon attending to mundane things." John le Carré wrote his first three novels during a ninety-minute commute to work; an occasional working lunch or evening burst brought his average up to four or five hours daily. Patrick O'Brian would start work "after breakfast and work or ponder until lunch," take the afternoon off, then look over his work between tea and dinnertime. The science fiction writer J. G. Ballard described his daily routine as "two hours in the late morning, two in the early afternoon, followed by a walk along the river to think over the next day." Chicago-based playwright Laura Schellhardt advises writers to "spend three or four hours a day, four or five days a week, in a room with your computer, your characters, and your plot." Screenwriters Syd Field—best known for his 1979 book *Screenplay*, a virtual bible for Hollywood writers—and Robert Towne, who won an Academy Award for *Chinatown*, wrote for four hours a day. Scott Adams, the creator of *Dilbert*, works about four hours a day on the strip and other writing; as he points out, "My value is based on my best ideas in any given day, not the number of hours I work." Stephen King describes four to six hours of reading and writing as a "strenuous" day. When it opened in 1954, the Center for Advanced Study in the Behavioral Sciences, located in the hills just above Stanford University, imagined a visiting fellow's ideal day as a morning working in monastic solitude from eight thirty to noon in two ninety-minute bursts with two fifteen-minute breaks, followed by lunch and an afternoon of walks and conversation. Even more volcanic artistic personalities can fall into a four-hour pattern. Arthur Koestler was a notorious drinker and womanizer, yet he settled into his desk for four hours every morning, with an occasional second session in the afternoon. Koestler developed this discipline while living rough in Palestine in the 1920s, and even in occupied France in the spring of 1940, when, his wife Daphne recalled, he rushed to finish *Darkness at Noon* before being discovered by the Nazis, he worked "with concentrated fury" until lunch, then returned to their flat for a couple more hours' writing.

The pattern of working four hard hours with occasional breaks isn't just confined to scientists, writers, or other people who are already successful, well-established, and have the freedom to set their own schedules. You can also see it among students who go on to become leaders in their fields. As a law student, young Thomas Jefferson balanced reading, attending court sessions, and assisting his teacher George Wythe with cases. Jefferson had previously followed a punishing schedule as a student, starting at dawn and reading into the night, but he discovered "a great inequality" in the "vigor of the mind at different times of day." As a law student he reserved four hours in the morning for intensive reading of law textbooks like Littleton's *English Law* and Coke's *Institutes of the Laws of England*. After lunch, he would read politics. A two-mile run or ride would follow in the afternoon, weather permitting. William Osler, who created the first residency program for training doctors while a professor at Johns Hopkins University School of Medicine, advised students to work "four or five hours daily," so long as they were hours "directed intensely upon the subject in hand."

This four-hour schedule was one serious Oxford and Cambridge students followed during reading parties in the 1800s and early 1900s. The academic calendars at the ancient universities feature several long vacations, and as one student wrote, in the spring a serious student "[gave] up the bulk of his long vacation to hard, methodical study," usually with a few friends and a hired tutor. The more scenic parts of England and Scotland were popular destinations, though parties also took over Alpine inns and lodges in the Black Forest. Once settled, Cambridge professor Karl Breul recalled, students would "work in the morning, and sometimes also in the evening, while the whole afternoon is given up to excursions or any kind of exercise amid pleasant surroundings." Even the more diligent students believed that once removed from the distractions of college life, they only needed a hard morning's work to "get through as much reading as we should have done at Oxford in half a term."

KARL ANDERS ERICSSON, Ralf Krampe, and Clemens Tesch-Römer saw a similar pattern in a study of violin students at a conservatory in Berlin in the 1980s. Ericsson, Krampe, and Tesch-Römer were interested in what sets outstanding students apart from merely good ones. After interviewing music students and their teachers and having students keep track of their time, they found that several things separated the best students from the rest.

First, the great students didn't just practice more than the average, they practiced more deliberately. During deliberate practice, Ericsson explained, you're "engaging with full concentration in a special activity to improve one's performance." You're not just doing reps, lobbing balls, or playing scales. Deliberate practice is focused, structured, and offers clear goals and feedback; it requires paying attention to what you're doing and observing how you can improve. Students can engage in deliberate practice when they have a clear route to greatness, defined by a shared understanding of what separates brilliant work from good work, or winners from losers. Endeavors where one can have the fastest time, the highest score, or the most elegant solution are ones that allow for deliberate practice.

Second, you need a reason to keep at it, day after day. Deliberate practice isn't a lot of fun, and it's not immediately profitable. It means being in the pool before sunrise, working on your swing or stride when you could be hanging out with friends, practicing fingering or breathing in a windowless room, spending hours perfecting details that only a few other people will ever notice. There's little that's inherently or immediately pleasurable in deliberate practice, so you need a strong sense that these long hours will pay off, and that you're not just improving your career prospects but also crafting a professional and personal identity. You don't just do it for the fat stacks. You do it because it reinforces your sense of who you are and who you will become.

The idea of deliberate practice and Ericsson et al.'s measurements of the total amount of time world-class performers spend practicing have received a lot of attention. The study is a foundation for Malcolm Gladwell's argument (laid out most fully in his book *Outliers*) that ten thousand hours of practice are necessary to become world-class in anything, and that everyone from chess legend Bobby Fischer to Microsoft founder Bill Gates to the Beatles put in their ten thousand hours before anyone heard of them. For coaches, music teachers, and ambitious parents, the number promises a golden road to the NFL or Juilliard or MIT: just start them young, keep them busy, and don't let them give up. In a culture that treats stress and overwork as virtues rather than vices, ten thousand hours is an impressively big number.

But there was something else that Ericsson and his colleagues noted in their study, something that almost everyone has subsequently overlooked. "Deliberate practice," they observed, "is an effortful activity that can be sustained only for a limited time each day." Practice too little and you never become world-class. Practice too much, though, and you increase the odds of being struck down by injury, draining yourself mentally, or burning out. To succeed, students must "avoid exhaustion" and "limit practice to an amount from which they can completely recover on a daily or weekly basis."

How do students marked for greatness make the most of limited practice time? The rhythm of their practice follows a distinctive pattern. They put in more hours per week in the practice room or playing field, but they don't do it by making each practice longer. Instead, they have more frequent, shorter sessions, each lasting about eighty to ninety minutes, with half-hour breaks in between.

Add these several practices up, and what do you get? About four hours a day. About the same amount of time Darwin spent every day doing his hardest work, Jefferson spent reading the law, Hardy and Littlewood spent doing math, Dickens and Koestler spent writing. Even ambitious young students in one of the world's best schools, preparing for an notoriously competitive field, could handle only four hours of really focused, serious effort per day.

This upper limit, Ericsson concluded, is defined "not by available time, but by available [mental and physical] resources for effortful practice." The students weren't just practicing four hours and calling it a day; lectures, rehearsals, homework, and other things kept them busy the rest of the day. In interviews, the students said "it was primarily their ability to sustain the concentration necessary for deliberate practice that limited their hours of practice." This is why it takes a decade to get Gladwell's ten thousand hours: if you can only sustain that level of concentrated practice for four hours a day, that works out to twenty hours a week (assuming weekends off), or a thousand hours a year (assuming a two-week vacation).

It's not just the lives of musicians that illustrate the importance of deliberate practice. Ray Bradbury began writing seriously in 1932 and wrote a thousand words a day. "For ten years I wrote at least one short story a week," he recalled, but they never quite came together. Finally, in 1942, he wrote "The Lake." Years later he still remembered the moment.

"Ten years of doing everything wrong suddenly became the right idea, the right scene, the right characters, the right day, the right creative time. I wrote the story sitting outside, with my typewriter, on the lawn. At the end of an hour the story was finished, the hair on the back of my neck was standing up, and I was in tears. I knew I had written the first really good story of my life."

Ericsson and his colleagues observed another thing, in addition to practicing more, that separated the great students at the Berlin Conservatory from the good, something that has almost been completely ignored since: how they rested.

The top performers actually slept about an hour a day more than the average performers. They didn't sleep late. They got more sleep because they napped during the day. Of course there was lots of variability, but the best students generally followed a pattern of practicing hardest and longest in the morning, taking a nap in the afternoon, and then having a second practice in the late afternoon or evening.

The researchers also asked students to estimate the amount of time they spent practicing, studying, and so on, and then had them keep a diary for a week. When they compared results from interviews and diaries, they noticed a curious anomaly in the data.

The merely good violinists tended to underestimate the amount of time they spent in leisure activities: they guessed they spent about fifteen hours a week, when in reality they spent almost twice that. The best violinists, in contrast, could "estimate quite accurately the time they allocated to leisure," about twenty-five hours. The best performers devoted more energy to organizing their time, thinking about how they would spend their time, and assessing what they did.

In other words, the top students were applying some of the habits of deliberate practice—mindfulness, an ability to observe their own performance, a sense that their time was valuable and needed to be spent wisely—to their downtime.

Nearly a century ago, music psychologist Carl Emil Seashore advised students, "The command to rest is fully as important as to work in effective learning." Rest and intensive practice, he said, worked together: practicing at your peak abilities for shorter periods, rather than halfheartedly throughout the day, "not only saves time in learning but develops those traits of personality in which you show yourself master of the situation." The top performers at the Berlin conservatory discovered this for themselves. They were spending fewer hours per day in leisure activity than their less-ambitious friends. But they kept better track of their leisure hours, which suggests that they were also more mindful about what they did with their time. They were putting in longer hours and practicing harder, and in order to keep up this schedule, they were using their leisure time more effectively.

They were discovering the immense value of deliberate rest. They figured out early that rest is important, that some of our most creative work happens when we take the kinds of breaks that allow our unconscious minds to keep plugging away, and that we can learn how to rest better. In the conservatory, deliberate rest is the partner of deliberate practice. It is in the studio and laboratory and publishing house, too. As Dickens and Poincaré and Darwin discovered, each is necessary. Each is half of a creative life. Together they form a whole.

For all the attention the Berlin conservatory study has received, this part of the top students' experiences—their sleep patterns, their attention to leisure, their cultivation of deliberate rest as a necessary complement of demanding, deliberate practice—goes unmentioned. In *Outliers*, Malcolm Gladwell focuses on the number of hours exceptional performers practice and says nothing about the fact that those students also slept an hour more, on average, than their less-accomplished peers, or that they took naps and long breaks.

This is not to say that Gladwell misread Ericsson's study; he just glossed over that part. And he has lots of company. Everybody speed-reads through the discussion of sleep and leisure and argues about the ten thousand hours.

This illustrates a blind spot that scientists, scholars, and almost all of us share: a tendency to focus on focused work, to assume that the road to greater creativity is paved by life hacks, propped up by eccentric habits, or smoothed by Adderall or LSD. Those who research world-class performance focus only on what students do in the gym or track or practice room. Everybody focuses on the most obvious, measurable forms of work and tries to make those more effective and more productive. They don't ask whether there are other ways to improve performance, and improve your life.

This is how we've come to believe that world-class performance comes after 10,000 hours of practice. But that's wrong. It comes after 10,000 hours of deliberate practice, 12,500 hours of deliberate rest, and 30,000 hours of sleep.

Morning Routine

It is wonderful how much work can be got through in a day, if we go by the rule—map out our time, divide it off, and take up one thing regularly after another. To drift through our work, or to rush through it in a helter-skelter fashion, ends in comparatively little being done. "One thing at a time" will always perform a better day's work than doing two or three things at a time. By following this rule, one person will do more in a day than another does in a week.

—Thomas Mitchell, *Essays on Life*

Every morning at 5 a.m., Scott Adams wakes up and heads downstairs to his kitchen, has a cup of coffee and a protein bar for breakfast, then goes into his home office. By 5:10 he's settled into his chair and working on his first task of the day: a new strip of *Dilbert*, the comic strip he's been drawing for almost thirty years. *Dilbert* began running in newspapers when Adams was an engineer working at Pacific

Bell; back then, he had to get up at 4 a.m. to write. ("That's why I rarely drew background scenery," he once explained. "I literally didn't have the time.") By 1995 *Dilbert* was doing well enough for him to become a full-time comic strip artist and to start expanding the *Dilbert* empire: *The Joy of Work*, his first nonfiction business book, came out in 1996. Still, he kept up his morning routine, and the morning hours are still when Adams gets most of his work done.

As he gets more deeply into the work, he notices, "Time passes differently when you are in the creative mindset. The first four hours of my day"—there are those four hours again!—"pass as though minutes." By then, if all goes well, he'll have finished a couple strips, blog posts, and tweets, and handled some correspondence or paperwork. An hour later, "the creativity well starts to run dry." By lunchtime, it's time for the gym. At that point, "my barely functioning brain is ideally suited for lifting heavy objects and putting them right back where I found them."

Adams is famous for making comic hay of the absurdities of corporate life and all the obstacles that get in the way of real creative work. So it's not surprising that his own early-morning routine is designed to avoid creative impediments, to let him get work done while the world is still asleep, and that it's well-thought-out and consistent. The coffee and protein bar? "The tastes are amazing together," he says, it prevents him being distracted later by hunger, and it's allowed him "to enjoy waking up and being productive." There are no variations in this routine. Setting "my physical body on autopilot for the morning . . . frees my brain for creativity."

He purposely excludes external stimulation. "My morning is all about stilling the outside world so my mind can soar." Like many writers, he keeps this routine because creativity "is not something you can summon on command," he says. "The best you can do is set an attractive trap and wait. My mornings are the trap."

It's not just stable from morning to morning. Adams was interviewed about his working style when *Dilbert* was first taking off; almost twenty years later, in 2014, he wrote a long essay about how he "engineers" his morning routine. A few details had changed over the years, but the essentials stayed the same. Adams's morning routine started as a necessity, a way to produce *Dilbert* without giving up his regular job, but over the years it's become a way to help his best ideas come to light. Working this way, he's turned *Dilbert* into a media empire: the strip appears in two thousand newspapers in sixty-five countries (and in twenty-five languages) and has spun out five books of cartoons, nine nonfiction books, a short-lived television show, and a movie project.

Adams's schedule illustrates two features of the working days of creatives who discover the power of deliberate rest: it starts early, and it follows a well-thought-out routine. Some writers and artists and scientists burn the midnight oil, depend on a looming deadline to help them focus, or wait for inspiration to strike before putting pen to paper. They accept that inspiration is unpredictable, creativity is unavoidably messy, and great work requires sacrifice and working under pressure. In contrast, many creatives who have long, productive careers take a different approach and attitude. They start work earlier, sometimes before dawn, even if they're night owls rather than early risers. They concentrate on their most challenging work first, when their creative energy is likely to be at its peak. They believe in inspiration but don't wait for it; instead, they find that work creates the conditions for inspiration. And they discover that rest improves rather than inhibits their creativity and can make them more productive, not less. Developing and maintaining a morning routine creates space in the day for rest, and makes rest more valuable.

I argued earlier that the world does not give us time for rest, that we have to take it. The early start makes room in the day for rest. It gives us the right to rest. It can also boost your creativity during those working hours and prime your subconscious mind to keep working even when you turn your attention to other things.

ADAMS MAKES SURE that "the first creative energy I spend of the day" is on the comic. Such an orderly, workmanlike attitude may not sound like a formula for creativity, but it's very common.

Among corporate leaders and finance types, an early start is a regular feature of daily life. Some jump into work immediately. For executives running multinational corporations or working in global financial markets, an early morning is a necessity because international markets are operating around the clock. The first e-mails of the day from Apple CEO Tim Cook go out around 4:30 a.m. California time, and by five he's working out. When he was running the investment firm Pimco, Bill Gross would wake up at 4:30 a.m. Pacific time (lunchtime in the London markets and early afternoon in Frankfurt). According to a 2014 survey by *Quartz*, 44 percent of executives check the news (these days, often reading on their smartphones) first thing in the morning. For other executives, an early rise gives them a chance to exercise. Hans Vestberg, CEO of Swedish telecommunications company Ericsson, rises early to run or work out at the gym. Jack Dorsey, the CEO of Twitter and Square, wakes up at five thirty to meditate and run. By then, Starbucks's Howard Schultz has already been up an hour and has finished his morning bike ride. Xerox CEO and chairwoman Ursula Burns rises before six and works out with a personal trainer twice a week. Frits van Paasschen, formerly CEO of Starwood Hotels and Resorts (they own the Sheraton and Westin chains, among others), goes for a run at the relatively late hour of 6 a.m. but makes up for it by running ten miles.

For creative workers, in contrast, the dominant pattern is to wake up and get right to work. Architect Frank Lloyd Wright would wake up at four o'clock in the morning, work for three hours, then go back to sleep. After he became a full-time writer, John le Carré would start writing between four thirty and five o'clock in the morning. Ernest Hemingway and John Cheever, to name but two, started writing around dawn. Anthony Trollope paid a servant an extra five pounds a year to make his coffee and wake him up at 5:00 a.m. so he could write for three hours before going to his job at the post office. He later declared, "I owe more to him than to any one else for the success I have had." Maya Angelou would "rent a hotel room for a few months, leave my home at six, and try to be at work by six-thirty," writing until lunchtime. The elderly Paul Cézanne would paint from six o'clock to ten thirty each morning and again in the late afternoon. Some authors discover the virtues of focused mornings the hard way. When he first started writing fiction, Gabriel García Márquez tried writing all day but soon found "what I did in the afternoon had to be done over again the next morning." Focusing on his writing in the mornings helped him complete his masterpiece, *One Hundred Years of Solitude*.

While their schedules tend to be more constrained by classes and calendars, scientists are often early risers. Arnold Sommerfeld, a mathematician and theoretical physicist who trained some of the twentieth century's greatest physicists, insisted that serious science required an early morning start. When he was a student of Sommerfeld's, Werner Heisenberg (a future Nobel laureate) recalled, Wolfgang Pauli (another future Nobel laureate) would roll into the lab around noon. "Well, this is a mistake," Sommerfeld told him. "You do not work well at night; you work very much better early in the morning. So I think tomorrow morning you will come at eight o'clock to the Institute." Hans Selye, the father of the scientific study of stress and author of numerous books and fifteen hundred articles, did his most serious thinking and writing early in the morning. As a medical student, Selye got into the habit of getting up at six; as a professor at the University of Montreal, he would be at his office at the International Institute of Stress by six thirty, giving himself two hours to think deeply before the lab opened at eight thirty.

For many, the aim is not to shake off sleep quickly and start work but to ease their way from a state of dreaming to wakefulness. Selye would allow himself a half hour's "conversation . . . between my conscious and unconscious self" before getting out of bed. The Irish writer Edna O'Brien felt herself "nearer to the unconscious, the source of inspiration" in the morning. I discovered this myself a few years ago. As a student I burned lots of midnight oil, but once I had a job and children, I struggled to muster the energy to write at night. So I tried getting up before dawn and writing before anyone else in the house was up. To my surprise, not only did I have more time to write, the words came more easily: I was less prone to self-distraction and had just enough energy and awareness to write. After a couple weeks I discovered that if the night before I programmed the coffee machine, outlined the next morning's writing task, and even set out my clothes and queued up music to work to, I could, like Adams, put my body on automatic and focus even more tightly on writing.

Many writers believe they are more creative in the mornings, agreeing with Mario Vargas Llosa that "the early hours of the day . . . are the most creative hours." It turns out that scientists have been able to validate their intuition. Especially for night owls like me, they find, working in the early mornings can boost your creativity.

For years, psychologists have been interested in what they call inhibition, the ability to suppress task-irrelevant thoughts. This kind of inhibition is important for staying focused, especially when doing jobs that aren't inherently fascinating: you don't want an air traffic controller with low inhibition. But as researchers have also shown, lower inhibition can lead to increased creativity (think back to the work of Naama Mayseless and instances of paradoxical functional facilitation). When people feel most alert and active, their inhibition is highest; when they're low-energy and need a nap, their inhibition lowers. This suggests that people might be more creative during the low points in their daily circadian rhythm (the natural twenty-four-hour cycle that governs energy levels, hormones, and other bodily functions). Psychologists Mareike Wieth and Rose Zacks set out to test whether circadian rhythm and tiredness affect problem-solving, insight, and imagination. They designed a test with three insight problems and three analytic problems and divided 428 undergraduates randomly into two groups. One group took the test in the morning, while the other took it in the late afternoon. After completing the test, subjects filled out a questionnaire about sleep habits and other preferences that revealed their chronotype, whether they were morning people or evening people.

When they analyzed the results, Wieth and Zacks found that student performance on the analytic portion of the test didn't vary with circadian rhythm or chronotype: students did equally well near their optimal circadian peak and during nonoptimal times. On the other hand, "insight problem solving was consistently greater at a participants' non-optimal time of day": early birds did better on the insight questions in the late afternoon, during their circadian lows, while night owls produced more insights in the morning, when their circadian rhythm was low.

One potential problem to working outside your circadian peak is that you're more easily distracted. However, a study by University of Arizona psychologist Cynthia May found that under the right circumstances, this effect can be turned to your advantage. May was interested in the relationship between people's problem-solving abilities, distractibility, and circadian rhythms. She placed subjects in front of a computer screen and gave them a Remote Associates Test: the screen displayed three words for thirty seconds, and they had to come up with a fourth word that connected all three. Occasionally, a distractor word also appeared on the screen; even though it was within their field of view, subjects were told to ignore it and focus only on the test words. In reality, though, some of the distractor words were misleading while others were actually helpful. (For example, if the three words were *helium, trial,* and *weather,* the correct answer would be *balloon.* A misleading distractor might be *chemistry,* while a leading distractor would be *floating.*) May hypothesized that when people were at their circadian peak, they would have an easier time pushing the distractors out of their minds and focusing only on the test words. In off-peak times, though, subjects would be more influenced by the distractors: they'd get fewer answers right when shown a misleading distractor and more right when shown a leading distractor.

May ran the test on two groups, college-age students in their teens and twenties and retirees in their sixties and seventies. What she found was that during off-peak times, the distractors had a big impact on performance—but for both groups, the leading distractors had a bigger influence than the misleading distractors. In other words, "when distracting material was related to task goals, individuals actually benefited from reduced inhibitory efficiency."

It's a bit of a jump from this kind of experiment to the real world, but the results suggest that there are "situations in which individuals are able to benefit from impaired inhibition," May concluded. Some early-morning creative workers take advantage of this effect. Hans Selye's early morning office, for example, was a space that surrounded him with "helpful" distractions like journal articles, books, and notes and insulated him from the "misleading" distractors of students and administrative duties. Writers and composers who shut themselves in their studies in the early morning are likewise creating environments rich in helpful distractions at a time when their creative minds are more likely to be responsive to them and better able to use them to form new associations and insights.

Even if you're not a night owl getting a creative high by working during your circadian lows, an early morning start has practical benefits. It can be a way of getting creative work done before the world has a chance to intrude. Nobel Prize–winning author Isaac Bashevis Singer lamented, "I am all the time interrupted" during the day, and writing in the early morning was his way to create undistracted time. For Toni Morrison, "Writing before dawn began as a necessity": when she was working on *The Bluest Eye*, *Sula*, and *Song of Solomon* in the 1970s, she was raising two children and working as an editor, and the pre-dawn hours were the only time she could write undisturbed. Later, when writing *Beloved*, the "habit of getting up early . . . became my choice," she said; "I realized that I was clearer-headed, more confident and generally more intelligent in the morning."

An early start also opens space in your day for rest and allows you to establish a clean division between working and resting time. One should "either work all out or rest completely," Cambridge mathematician John Littlewood advised. Even for people whose minds naturally gravitate to their work, having clear boundaries between periods of work and rest allows them to get more from each. "It is too easy, when rather tired, to fritter a whole day away with the intention of working but never getting properly down to it," Littlewood said. "This is pure waste, nothing is done, and you have had no rest or relaxation." Virtually every prolific author and scientist would agree. A day that starts with work creates rest that can be enjoyed without guilt. When you start early, the rest you take is the rest you've earned.

CREATIVE PEOPLE WHO discover deliberate rest don't just spend a few focused hours each day working or prefer to concentrate their effort in the morning. They work the same hours of the day, every day, often seven days a week. Stephen King exemplifies the attitude that routine is critical to creative production. He hasn't written dozens of books in transcendent, days-long blazes. King works methodically, he explains in *On Writing*, putting in "four to six hours a day, every day." Writing, he says, is "just another job like laying pipe or driving long-haul trucks." Just as a regular bedtime helps you sleep better, a regular daily schedule—"in at about the same time every day, out when your thousand words are on paper or disk—exists in order to habituate yourself, to make yourself ready to dream just as you make yourself ready to sleep."

For King and other prolific creatives, this kind of routine doesn't impede creativity but supports it. "Routine becomes invaluable to writers," said Tobias Wolff, the author of *This Boy's Life* and *In Pharaoh's Army*. William Osler advised students that "four or five hours daily it is not much to ask" to devote to their studies, "but one day must tell another, one week certify another, one month bear witness to another of the same story." A few hours haphazardly spent and giant bursts of effort were both equally fruitless; it was necessary to combine focus and routine. (He lived what he preached: one fellow student recalled that in his habits Osler was "more regular and systematic than words can say.")

Anthony Trollope dismissed the idea that writers had to wait for inspiration or that genius was unpredictable. He advised writers to "avoid enthusiastic rushes with their pens, and to seat themselves at their desks day by day as though they were lawyers' clerks." Trollope kept to his routine by keeping a diary with a daily writing schedule for each book and tracking how many words he had written each day, "so that if at any time I have slipped into idleness for a day or two, the record of that idleness has been there, staring me in the face, and demanding of me increased labour." Just as

William James argued in "The Gospel of Relaxation" that a steady emotional state is less wearying and more productive than grand displays of passion, Trollope advised that a "small daily task, if it be really daily, will beat the labours of a spasmodic Hercules." Raymond Chandler, whose hard-boiled detectives cast a long shadow across modern mystery writing, said that "there should be a space of time, say four hours a day at the least, when a professional writer doesn't do anything but write." You don't have to write during those hours, Chandler added, but you can't do anything else.

But what if you aren't inspired? Ingmar Bergman said that it is necessary to "sit down pedantically every day at a definite time, irrespective of whether you're in the mood or not." Tchaikovsky believed that "a self-respecting artist must not fold his hands on the pretext that he is not in the mood." Joyce Carol Oates agreed: "One must be pitiless about this matter of 'mood'" and start writing no matter what; "the writing will create the mood." Trollope ridiculed the idea that "the man who works with his imagination should allow himself to wait till—inspiration moves him." As far as he was concerned, "it would not be more absurd if the shoemaker were to wait for inspiration."

The reason it's necessary to start writing, and to keep writing, is that creativity doesn't drive the work; the work drives creativity. A routine creates a landing place for the muse. Stephen King believes in the importance of the muse, but his muse isn't an ethereal character who comes "flitting down into your writing room and scatter creative fairy-dust all over your typewriter." King's muse is "a basement guy" who "sits and smokes cigars and admires his bowling trophies" while "you do all the grunt work." He's stubborn and difficult to please. But the creative world waits on him, and he knows it. Why? Because "the guy with the cigar and the little wings has got a bag of magic," and everyone knows that "there's stuff in there that can change your life." But you've got to earn it. Do the work, "make sure the muse knows where you're going to be every day from nine to noon or seven to three," and "sooner or later he'll start showing up, chomping his cigar and making his magic."

We think of routine as the opposite of creativity: things done by routine require little thought and leave no room for creative interpretation or flexibility. In reality, German sociologists Sandra Ohly, Sabine Sonnentag, and Franziska Pluntke argue, routines can enhance creativity. They surveyed three hundred workers at a German high-tech company about how much routine there was in their everyday work, how much opportunity they had to be creative on the job, and how much initiative they could exercise in trying out new ideas. They then looked at rates of contribution to an in-house program that solicited suggestions for manufacturing improvements, new products, and so on. They found that employees whose work had a large measure of routine were more likely to submit ideas. By this measure, they were more creative.

When the researchers dug into the numbers, they noticed something else: employees who exhibited more creativity had jobs with a higher proportion of routine, but they also had more control over their work. Their daily work consisted of tasks they could learn to do automatically, but because they could choose how to organize their work, they became more reflective about how things worked, better able to notice how they might be improved, and more likely to feel able to make suggestions. Routinization of work, the researchers concluded, does not have to diminish creativity; if it's accompanied by freedom, routine can enhance creativity.

Other studies have found similar positive relationships between routine and creativity and help us understand how they can work together. Shared routines can help groups work better. Routines don't tap into willpower, resilience, or intrinsic motivation, leaving you more of those resources to spend on hard problems. Routines also save time and energy. A writer who's fluent in a language and can touch-type can focus on developing her argument or unfolding a mystery; she doesn't have to labor over how to spell words or search around the keyboard for a letter. When they take physical form, routines can support fast, creative action. Professional chefs and line cooks, for example, put lots of energy into assembling their mise-en-place, the implements, ingredients, spices and sauces they'll need during their shift. Like a hiker's pack or a doctor's surgical tray, the mise-en-place should have everything a cook needs to deal with any situation, organized for effortless retrieval. Indeed, chefs describe the mise-en-place as both a physical organization and a state of mind, and teach that the one supports the other: having all tools and ingredients in exactly the right place lets chefs get into that state of flow that permits them to work quickly and at a high level. Routines can also provide just enough pressure to stimulate creativity but not so much that they inhibit creativity. Small, self-imposed daily goals, like Trollope's word count, seem to stimulate concentration and prod creativity but aren't make-or-break: when your habit is to work steadily, a day when you fall behind isn't fatal.

A COMBINATION OF routine and freedom, a world laid out to support creative work while reducing unnecessary distractions and peripheral decisions, nicely describes the world that focused mornings and routines make. And if creativity is supported by routine, rest is absolutely dependent on it. Each is easily crowded out by the day's noise, by regular demands and distractions, and by unexpected emergencies or opportunities. In order to keep rest from being invaded by work or crowded out of your day by a long to-do list, you need to use your routine like a fortification to protect your time. That same routine also lets you get more done and makes you more creative. It's another example of how work and rest are subtly connected and mutually reinforcing.

Creative people don't get up early to work, labor steadily rather than spasmodically, and follow a strict schedule so they can take it easy the rest of the day. They think about their work constantly, but by organizing their days around early starts and regular hours, they don't have to rely on their conscious minds. For them, early mornings and routines set the flywheel of the unconscious spinning. As Stephen King puts it, a routine will "train your waking mind to sleep creatively and work out the vividly imagined waking dreams which are successful works of fiction." Their afternoons may be spent doing more mundane tasks, but they're able to do more, and do better work, because they use routines, concentrated periods of focused work, and periods of deliberate rest, rather than long hours of labor. For some, the early morning lets them play against their circadian rhythms, dampening the influence of the brain's evaluative system, lowering inhibition, and stimulating creativity. An early start also creates space in the day for rest.

You need time for rest because that's when the unconscious mind can get to work. You can't command inspiration to appear, but you can nudge it, most notably by working steadily and regularly. The romantic image of the artist who does nothing until he's inspired and then produces in a furious burst of work is misleading. For Henri Poincaré, who studied his own creative process pretty carefully, it seemed that the flash of insight—what he called illumination—only occurs "if it is on the one hand preceded and on the other hand followed by a period of conscious work." As Pablo Picasso said, "Inspiration exists, but it has to find you working." Or as illustrator Chuck Close put it, "Inspiration is for amateurs. The rest of us just show up and get to work."

Late in life, Anthony Trollope explained what allowed him to be so productive. Even while he held down a full-time job, over a writing career that stretched more than forty years, he published forty-seven novels and sixteen volumes of nonfiction (more than a book a year), as well "political articles, critical, social, and sporting articles, for periodicals, without number." Despite this amazing output, he went hunting twice weekly, "lived much in society in London," regularly entertained friends at Waltham Cross, and "always spent six weeks at least out of England. Few men, I think, ever lived a fuller life. And I attribute the power of doing this altogether to the virtue of early hours."

Walk

It is quite nice to have an office and even nicer
to have a warm, well-furnished home. But my
mind often comes to a standstill after some hours
indoors. So I take a walk. Once outside, my mind
immediately begins to move freely and instinctively
over my subject. Ideas come rushing to my mind,
without being called. Soon enough, the best answer
emerges from the jumble. I realize what I can do,
what I should do, and what I must abandon.

—Eugene Wigner

"I HAVE WALKED MYSELF into my best thoughts," declared
the Danish philosopher Søren Kierkegaard. Kierkegaard was famous for his long walks through Copenhagen,
but he could be speaking for many philosophers, and for
everyone who practices deliberate rest. Walking and thinking have been amiable companions since ancient times. The
connection is reflected in the fact that we refer to members

of a philosophical school as "followers." It's expressed in the phrase *solvitur ambulando* ("it is solved by walking"), variously attributed to the Greek philosopher Diogenes, Saint Augustine, and other ancient and medieval thinkers. Walking is a great example of a natural activity that we can learn to adapt to new purposes. Among creative thinkers, it provides time to clear the mind or get a fresh perspective on a problem. It can be solitary or social, a chance for conversation with one's self or with others. It can get you out of the office or be a mobile meeting.

For many thinkers and doers, a walk is an essential part of their daily routine, a source of exercise and solitude. Thomas Jefferson advised his nephew to walk for mental relaxation and for physical endurance and added, "Never think of taking a book with you. The object of walking is to relax the mind [and] divert your attention by the objects surrounding you." Jefferson practiced what he preached, walking in the mornings before breakfast "to shake off sleep," taking five-mile tramps around Paris during his posting as ambassador, and, as president, reserving time during the afternoon for walking or riding. As a student preparing for his entrance examinations to Oxford, C. S. Lewis got into the habit of taking an afternoon walk after a long morning studying. Such walks were occasions for contemplation, not conversation: "Walking and talking are two very great pleasures," he wrote, "but it is a mistake to combine them." Graham Wallas, author of *The Art of Thought*, would walk several miles a day, as a break from writing and preparing lectures or to get his blood flowing after a long morning reading in the

British Library. The writer Alice Munro walks three miles every day. For Charles Dickens, "daily walks were less of rule than of enjoyment and necessity," one of his many biographers said. Dickens took long walks: ten or twelve miles was typical, and when he was troubled he might cover eighteen miles in an afternoon, often accompanied by one of his large, protective dogs, which was helpful when walking in the less savory parts of London. Three or four hours of walking a day sounds like a long time in a busy day, but "I could not keep my health otherwise," he said. Uber CEO Travis Kalanick walks forty miles a week on the indoor track at the company's San Francisco headquarters. That's a lot, particularly for someone who could just call for a car, but as business writer Tony Schwartz notes, many executives who are smart about maintaining their energy take afternoon walks to recharge.

Indeed, walking meetings have become popular, especially among Silicon Valley entrepreneurs and CEOs. It might seem odd that a region that has gotten rich from people spending unhealthily long hours at their desks would take to walking meetings as enthusiastically as bespoke hoodies or electric cars, but as one executive points out, "most of a software engineer's job is not about physically writing code; it is about solving problems, thinking, discussing, bouncing ideas off each other," and walking meetings can be good for all of those things. Steve Jobs was famous for his walking meetings around the leafy streets of Palo Alto. At LinkedIn, employees frequently take to the bike and walking paths in Shoreline Park, just outside the company's headquarters; Google's Mountain View campus is laced with walking paths.

Facebook's corporate headquarters in Menlo Park, California, designed by Frank Gehry and opened in early 2015, is a vast open-plan building (supposedly the world's largest) topped off with a nine-acre garden roof featuring a half-mile walking path. A few companies have mapped out thirty- and fifty-minute routes around their campuses and allow employees to reserve "walking meeting rooms" in company calendars and scheduling programs.

Ted Eytan, a physician who's medical director of the Kaiser Permanente Center for Total Health, has been a fan of walking meetings for more than a decade. The modern office makes us sit too much, he argues, which affects our cardiovascular health, weakens our bodies, and dulls our brains. During a walking meeting, Eytan notes, you get physical stimulation—a half hour's walk can provide a mile's or mile and a half's worth of exercise—but your brain is more active, too. Walking meetings, counterintuitively, can also be more private, especially if you work in an open office: a city street can shield you from eavesdroppers, and being away from colleagues will keep you from being interrupted. Some people find it easier to discuss personal or sensitive matters on a walk, partly because it's a more relaxed setting, without the uncomfortable intimacy of a one-on-one office meeting. A walking meeting also separates subordinates who need the certainty of PowerPoint decks and offices from those who can (literally) think on their feet.

There are particular benefits for executives. As Jeff Weiner notes, a walking meeting "essentially eliminates distractions, so I find it to be a much more productive way to spend time."

Like most executives', Weiner's working day at LinkedIn (where he's CEO) is pureed into tiny fragments of time: decades ago, management experts estimated that CEOs normally can only devote a couple minutes to a problem or task before they have to switch gears, and this was before e-mail. A walking meeting can provide a welcome opportunity to focus on one thing for more than a few minutes. Finally, walking meetings are an opportunity to turn on the charm or drive a hard bargain: Steve Jobs was especially good at using walks to win over reluctant allies, and Mark Zuckerberg reportedly goes on walks with prized recruits and founders of start-ups Facebook wants to acquire.

Perhaps the most important walking meeting in history took place in 1938, when Howard Florey and Ernst Chain decided to work on developing the antibiotic penicillin. World War I had demonstrated the need for drugs to counter infections that struck deep in wounds caused by machine guns, artillery, and chlorine gas. In the 1920s, scientists had discovered that bacteria possessed an arsenal of chemical weapons that they used on each other, and in 1928 Alexander Fleming had noted that the mold *Pencillium notatum* had powerful defenses against disease-causing bacteria. Florey and Chain wondered if those antibacterial agents could be synthesized and used for treating infections in humans. Florey's mentor, Charles Sherrington, had advised Florey to live far enough from the lab to get "sufficient exercise and out-of-door 'refresher' in passing to and fro," and he and Chain would brainstorm ideas for research projects while walking home through Oxford's University Parks.

Florey and Chain began working on penicillin in 1939; by 1941, they had demonstrated its efficacy on humans, and Allied governments took up mass production of the drug. By the end of the war, penicillin was rightly hailed for helping to save tens of thousands of lives, and their work earned Florey and Chain a share of the 1945 Nobel Prize in Physiology or Medicine, the first awarded after the war.

Others consciously use walking as a way of loosening creative inhibitions. For example, Nobel Prize–winning economist Herbert Simon used the mile-long walk from home to his office at Carnegie Mellon University as "thinking time," his daughter Katherine said. When they were working on the structure of DNA, James Watson and Francis Crick would regularly take walks around Cambridge after lunch, talk over the morning's work, and consider their next steps. When they were visitors at Stanford University in the late 1970s, Daniel Kahneman, Amos Tversky, and Richard Thaler would take long walks in the hills above the Center for Advanced Study in the Behavioral Sciences, exploring ideas that would eventually become the foundation of behavioral economics. The Russian composer Pyotr Ilyich Tchaikovsky would take a short walk in the morning before starting work and go out again for two hours in the afternoon. "Most of the time during these walks was spent in composition," his brother said. "He thought out the leading ideas, pondered over the construction of the work, and jotted down fundamental themes." Ludwig van Beethoven would take long afternoon walks in the woods around Vienna; he is said to have drawn inspiration from those walks when composing his Pastoral Symphony.

Composer Lin-Manuel Miranda wrote lyrics to *Hamilton* during long Sunday morning walks in the park with his dog, freestyling on top of beats or melodies he composed at home.

For physicists, walking offers a way to clear the mind without completely abandoning a problem. Eugene Wigner, who won a Nobel Prize in Physics for his work in nuclear and particle theory, was often seen wandering the Princeton campus. "My mind often comes to a standstill after some hours indoors," he said, but on a walk "my mind immediately begins to move freely and instinctively over my subject. Ideas come rushing to my mind, without being called. Soon enough, the best answer emerges from the jumble. I realize what I can do, what I should do, and what I must abandon." Theoretical physicist Paul Dirac, who at twenty-six was appointed the Lucasian Professor of Mathematics at Cambridge (the same professorship held by Isaac Newton, Charles Babbage, and Stephen Hawking), would take daylong walks on Sundays. "I would not intentionally think about my work" during those long walks, he said; "I found these occasions most profitable for new ideas."

The idea that walking relaxes and usefully diverts the mind received a boost from a study led by architect and neuroscientist Jenny Roe. She placed EEGs on the scalps of walkers in Edinburgh and recorded their brains' activity as they walked. When she examined the data, she found that she could tell from their brain waves when people were walking through parks and green space and when they were in busy commercial areas: their minds became calmer and less aroused when they turned from the high street into a park. They didn't zone out completely, though. Natural scenes engage some of our attention without requiring much conscious effort: they provide just enough diversion to occupy the conscious mind, leaving the subconscious free to do its own thing.

Sometimes walks don't just loosen inhibitions to creative thinking but also dislodge insights that have been working their way up from the subconscious. Geneticist Barbara McClintock identified the tiny chromosomes in the plant mold *Neurospora* during a long walk around the Stanford University campus filled with "very intense, subconscious thinking." When she suddenly visualized the answer—an answer that had eluded other geneticists for twenty years—"I jumped up, I couldn't wait to get back to the laboratory. I knew I was going to solve it." The nineteenth-century Irish mathematician William Rowan Hamilton literally carved his most famous insight, on the algebra of quaternions, on the bridge where it occurred while he was walking with his wife. An "under-current of thought was going on in my mind" as they walked along the Royal Canal, when suddenly "a spark flashed forth." In his account of the discovery of Fuchsian functions, the great French mathematician Henri Poincaré describes a series of a-ha moments that came while boarding a bus, on a walk on a seaside bluff near Caen, and walking down the street in Paris.

The uncertainty principle came to Werner Heisenberg during a late-night walk in Copenhagen in 1927. Heisenberg had been struggling with the fact that the equations he had developed could precisely predict the momentum of a particle but not its position. While walking in Fælled Park, he had an insight: what if there was no problem with the mathematics or the models? What if this uncertainty was actually a property of particles? Ernö Rubik made the critical design breakthrough that yielded the Rubik's Cube while walking along the River Danube. A teacher at the Academy of Applied Arts in Budapest, Rubik was trying to build a cube whose faces could rotate freely along all three axes. It was clear that the cube had to be made of smaller blocks, but he couldn't figure out how to hold them together. One spring day he went for a walk and was "looking at how the water moved around the pebbles" when the turbulence behind the pebbles inspired him to try a design in which the small blocks were held together with cantilevers on their corners or edges.

The sudden and unexpected nature of the insights make for dramatic stories, but a closer look reveals that all of these examples follow Wallas's model of preparation, incubation, and illumination. McClintock first encountered *Neurospora* years before her Stanford epiphany, and her illuminating walk came after a week of intensive work in the laboratory. Before his walk, Rubik had spent three months working on the problem, filling his apartment with hundreds of prototypes. Poincaré's insights on Fuchsian functions came in between months of false starts, hard work, and dead ends. Heisenberg had been working on the uncertainty problem for almost two years before his fateful walk in the park. Hamilton later wrote that the quaternions problem "had haunted me for at least fifteen years." In all these cases, long periods of preparation and incubation culminated in an unexpected moment of insight.

THERE IS AN obvious objection to the argument that walking stimulates creativity: that walking is so common an activity it's inevitable that some people would have moments of insight during them. The fact that Beethoven and Darwin took long daily walks, or that Rubik and McClintock had key insights during walks, doesn't mean that there is a relationship between walking and insight. After all, people report having sudden insights in the shower, too.

"One of the people on my committee actually asked, 'Why don't you run a condition in the shower?'" Stanford postdoc Marily Oppezzo says. "I told them, 'I can't get IRB [institutional review board] approval to study people when they shower.'" Oppezzo and education professor Daniel Schwartz published a widely cited article in 2014 on the effects of walking on creativity. Appropriately enough, the idea for the study first came when the two were taking a walk around campus and realized that while there was plenty of anecdotal evidence that walking stimulates creativity, no one had yet tried to measure it or figure out whether the stimulus came from walking itself, getting out of the office, being in nature, or some other factor.

Oppezzo and Schwartz designed four experiments that used standard psychological tools to measure creativity and could be done while walking. In the first experiment, students took two tests, Guilford's Alternative Uses Test (AUT), which measures creative divergent thinking, and the Compound Remote Associates Test (CRA), which measures convergent thinking. In the AUT, researchers measure how many alternative uses for a common object a subject can think of in a certain period, and how feasible those uses are. So, for example, if you were asked to come up with alternative uses for chopsticks, using them to prop up an iPad or hold down the pages of a book would score well on feasibility; using them as a spaceship would be imaginative but get a low feasibility rating. In the CRA, subjects are given three words (for example, *business, calling,* and *graphics,* or *cheese, school,* and *pine*) and have to come up with a fourth word that relates to each of them. (Think for a minute on those two examples.) The speed with which people are able to come up with an answer serves as a measure of how good they are at making or perceiving unlikely connections, which is one of the hallmarks of creativity. (The answers, by the way, are *card* and *board,* respectively.) Oppezzo and Schwartz chose these two tests because each highlights a different facet of creativity: the first is very open-ended and requires imagination, while the second requires coming up with a specific solution.

Oppezzo and Schwartz first had students take the AUT and CRA (in that order—if you take the CRA and do poorly, it inhibits your performance on subsequent tests) while sitting in a plain room. They all then got on a treadmill, found a comfortable walking pace, and took the AUT and CRA again (with different questions). It was actually important for the students to set the treadmill pace themselves, rather than have everyone walk at the same speed. "If you force somebody to walk at a pace that's not their own natural gait, it takes more attention," Oppezzo explains, "and your performance on certain tasks will go down."

The results were striking. In the first experiment, 81 percent of students did better on the AUT when walking on a treadmill than when sitting, but only 23 percent did better on the CRA. In fact, average scores on the CRA dropped slightly when students moved from sitting to walking. Indeed, many studies show that walking has a detrimental effect on tasks that require focused thinking and attention to detail. "It's not that we should all get treadmill desks and get on them all the time," Oppezzo says, "because it turns out it's probably only good for a couple types of thinking."

But maybe scores improved because people had a chance to practice, not because they were walking? In a second experiment, Oppezzo and Schwartz mixed things up. They had some students take the AUT while walking on the treadmill first, then when seated (the tread-sit group); others were tested while seated, then when on the treadmill (the sit-tread group); and a third group sat for both tests, to eliminate exercise as a factor on their performance (the sit-sit group).

Again, the results showed a striking relationship between exercise and creativity. The sit-sit group did a little worse the second time, suggesting that practice not only didn't improve scores, it had the opposite effect. Students in the sit-tread group got the same initial scores as the sit-sit group; when they got on the treadmill, their scores went way up. The really interesting results came from the tread-sit group. Their first responses were far more creative than those of the groups that started off sitting (on a scale from 0 to 15, they scored about 12, while the sitting groups scored about 4). When they sat down, the quality of their responses dropped a little (to about 9), but their second-round results were as good as those of the sit-tread group. In other words, walking had a dramatic initial impact on creativity and that effect remained strong, even when people sat down.

Oppezzo and Schwartz went outside for a third experiment. Treadmill desks may be a popular accessory among some hard-charging executives (though the metaphor of constantly moving and not getting anywhere seems more Charlie Chaplin than Charles Koch), but most of us walk by, well, walking around. So this time, they recruited another group of students (thankfully the Bay Area has lots of college students) and put them in four groups: sit-sit (both inside), sit (inside)-walk (outside), walk (outside)-sit (inside), and walk (outside)-walk (outside). This time, the sit-walk group experienced a dramatic increase in the novelty of their responses on the AUT, jumping from a mean of 4 to 10. The walk-sit group started high, then fell a bit (from 10 to 9), just as in the second experiment. The walk-walk group rose modestly, from 8 to 9.

And the sit-sit group? Their scored hovered between 4 and 5.

Finally, in a fourth experiment, Oppezzo and Schwartz again divided students into four groups. One group worked inside at a table (the SitIn group), one walked on a treadmill (WalkIn), one walked around campus (WalkOut), and one was pushed along the same campus path in a wheelchair (SitOut). Each group took a creativity test called the Symbolic Equivalence Test (SET), in which you come up with metaphors or equivalent images for a phrase like "windblown leaves" (test inventor Frank Barron suggested "a civilian population chaotically fleeing in the face of armed aggression" and "handkerchiefs being tossed about in an electric dryer" as equivalents).

Once again, the walkers scored higher than the sitters. But what was interesting about these results was that the treadmill walkers scored about the same as the outdoor walkers. The assumption that the gentle, low-level distractions of walking outdoors loosened the mind and allowed people to be more creative didn't explain why treadmill walkers, facing a blank wall, did as well on the SET—or why treadmill walkers outperformed people pushed outside in a wheelchair.

"We were surprised that we found the benefit in a bare room with construction sounds outside," Oppezzo admits. "The room was barely big enough for a desk and treadmill, and there were no windows, so we were stunned to see that effect." Like most of us, they had assumed that environment would play a larger role in stimulating creativity, that being in a pleasant environment rather than a cinder-block room would benefit people. This is how she and her adviser worked, after all, trading ideas while going for walks.

But it turned out that while students scored higher on the divergent-thinking test while walking outdoors than when they were sitting, and their outdoor walking scores were a lot higher than their scores sitting inside, their scores walking outdoors weren't really higher than their scores walking on a treadmill.

In other words, it isn't being outside that stimulates creativity; it is actually the walking itself that is most responsible for helping people be more creative.

So why does walking have this effect? Nobody is absolutely sure yet. "It could be mood, or maybe walking takes just enough focus that it lets seemingly irrelevant possibilities come to the forefront," Oppezzo says; or maybe walking "just allows more ideas to bubble up."

If you're still skeptical that creative people consciously incorporate walking into their creative lives, consider the fact that many of them are diligent about carrying notebooks when they walk. Many of Tchaikovsky's compositions began as notes jotted down in the forest and elaborated once he was back home. Beethoven carried paper and pencil on his long walks. For both men, writing while walking let them outline one idea, then put it safely aside and release their minds again to wander. Likewise, the physiologist Hans Selye carried a notebook to free his mind from the "information pollution" of small details and tasks and let him think about more serious subjects at "the limits of my tolerance." William Rowan Hamilton carried a "pocket-book" in which he could jot down ideas while on walks; so did Lin-Manuel Miranda while working on *Hamilton* lyrics during Sunday morning walks. The director Billy Wilder would carry a black notebook in which he wrote down ideas about dialogue, characters, and stories, some of which would make it into movies a decade later. *The Apartment*, for example, started as a quick note jotted down more than a decade earlier, after watching David Lean's *Brief Encounter*. "I always have a pencil with me, to the point where it forms a part of me," says Ferran Adrià, the great Spanish chef and father of molecular gastronomy. Even in the kitchen of his restaurant

El Bulli, where he was constantly on his feet, "I [was] always writing—taking notes, jotting down ideas," he says.

Even people who didn't carry notebooks came up with similar solutions for note-taking. The English political philosopher Thomas Hobbes walked with a cane that had an inkwell built into the handle and would write on a piece of paper attached to a board. The great German mathematician David Hilbert wrote down ideas as he walked but abandoned notebooks entirely: he installed a covered blackboard in his garden, and he and his assistants would make notes as he walked or worked in the flower beds.

Oppezzo and Schwartz's Stanford study and the work of Jenny Roe in Edinburgh show that the belief that walking stimulates creativity holds up to experimental verification. It's not great for focused, analytical thinking, and there's plenty left to be learned about the relationship between walking and creativity, but there are good reasons walking has been so large a part of the creative lives of philosophers, composers, writers, painters, and, more recently, innovation-seeking (and simply health-conscious) executives. Walking doesn't look like an intellectual activity, and there are plenty of times when it's purely utilitarian or recreational, but we can learn to use it to help us think better.

Most accounts of walking and thinking come from people who practiced it for years, and that's obscured the fact that we can actually learn to harness the benefits of walking. But a few accounts show that, like other forms of deliberate rest, walking for creativity involves skills that we can cultivate.

Barbara McClintock's experience illustrates that we can learn to use it. As a child, she told her biographer, she discovered that she could focus so deeply on activities that she'd lose her sense of self, to the point of forgetting her own name. As a graduate student, she learned to apply this ferocious capacity for attention to her scientific work and began to learn how to recognize when her subconscious was working through a problem. Her Stanford walk, she later said, was the first time she felt she had mastered the process. The *Neurospora* episode taught her that she could use walking to activate her unconscious, "to use it in the service of scientific discovery." Previously, McClintock said, this had worked episodically; after her time at Stanford, she claimed, she could "summon it when needed." Through a long career at Cold Spring Harbor, she would be renowned for her brilliance, for her ability to work for years on complicated projects, and for the long walks she would take while patiently working through problems. McClintock's ability to harness intuition on walks would help her make the revolutionary discovery of "jumping genes," sequences of DNA that move from one place to another in a chromosome, and help her win a Nobel Prize in Physiology or Medicine 1983. Like Kierkegaard, McClintock had learned to walk herself into her best thoughts.

Nap

I really nap a lot. Usually I get sleepy right after lunch, plop down on the sofa, and doze off. Thirty minutes later I come wide awake. As soon as I wake up, my body isn't sluggish and my mind is totally clear.

—Haruki Murakami

ONE OF THE more unlikely museums in London is located in the basement of the Treasury, between 10 Downing Street and the Palace of Westminster: the Churchill War Rooms, the underground complex from which Prime Minister Winston Churchill and his ministers and generals fought World War II. The War Rooms is a large warren of small offices, dormitories, and dining rooms for the prime minister and his staff, top cabinet officers, and general staff, hidden under a bomb-resistant five-foot-thick, steel-reinforced concrete ceiling. During World War II, hundreds of people worked in them, from clerks and secretaries to generals and ministers. Today, though, the space is dominated by the memory of Churchill. The exhibits describe the ups and downs of his political career; his indefatigable energy defending Britain and the empire; his eloquence and skill as a writer; his daily life during the war; and his mix of political opportunism, realpolitik, and idealism. But one aspect of his working life gets only a brief mention, at the end of the tour: his habit of taking daily naps.

Churchill himself regarded his midday naps as essential for maintaining his mental balance, renewing his energy, and reviving his spirits. He had gotten into the habit of napping during World War I, when he was First Lord of the Admiralty, and even during the Blitz Churchill would retire to his private room in the War Rooms after lunch, undress, and sleep for an hour or two. Unless German bombs were falling, he would then head to 10 Downing Street for a bath, change into fresh clothes, and return to work. Churchill's valet, Frank Sawyers, later recalled, "It was one of the inflexible rules of Mr. Churchill's daily routine that he should not miss this rest."

Not only did a nap help Churchill keep up his energy, his sangfroid also inspired his cabinet and officers. Napping during boring parliamentary debates was one thing. Going to sleep literally while bombs were falling signaled Churchill's confidence in his staff and his belief that the dark days would pass. Churchill wasn't the only Allied leader to nap regularly. George Marshall advised Dwight Eisenhower to take a daily nap; on the other side of the world, Pacific

Command adjusted its schedule around Douglas Mac-Arthur's afternoon nap, which was part of a daily schedule that "had scarcely changed since his days as superintendent of West Point," according to his biographer William Manchester. (Adolf Hitler, in contrast, kept more erratic hours at the best of times, and as the Allies closed in on Germany in 1944 and 1945, he tried to stay up for days at a time, powered by a mix of amphetamines, cocaine, and other drugs.)

Winston Churchill has been a model for many leaders, and at least two American presidents were inspired by his example to take up napping. John F. Kennedy was so "impressed by Churchill's eloquence in praise of the afternoon nap," said Arthur Schlesinger Jr., that when he entered the Senate he imitated Churchill's practice of keeping a cot in Parliament. Later at the White House, Kennedy would normally take a 45-minute nap after lunch; like Churchill, he wouldn't sleep in the office, but would head for the residence and change into pajamas. Kennedy's successor, Lyndon Johnson, likewise broke up his long day with a nap and shower in the afternoon. (The habit of lying down isn't just convenience: a Chinese sleep science lab measuring the effect of physical position on levels of sleepiness, fatigue, mood, and alertness found that people who napped lying down got more out of their naps than those who napped sitting up.)

A political figure may not seem creative, but politicians who lead during crises, generals who plan complex operations, and CEOs working in fast-changing industries need something of an artist's flexibility and insight. Governing a nation at war, holding together a far-flung empire against external threats and independence movements, negotiating with Roosevelt and Stalin, and juggling competing demands all required Churchill to display plenty of creativity. So it's no surprise that reserving time for a nap was one of Churchill's "inflexible rules." Creative people often become as attuned to their mental states as elite athletes are to their physical condition and energy levels. As a result, creative people who have to keep long hours and people whose demanding jobs require imagination and an ability to react, discover the restorative power of an afternoon nap. Sleep scientists have found that even a short nap can be effective in recharging your mental batteries. Naps can even provide an opportunity to have new ideas. Their work shows that you can learn to time your nap to increase the creative boost that it provides, make it more physically restorative, or probe the traffic between the conscious mind and unconscious. Napping, in other words, turns out to be a skill.

NAPS HAVE BEEN a part of the schedules of many creative people. When he was writing *The Martian Chronicles* in 1949, Ray Bradbury rented his parents' garage office a short bike ride from his home. He would work there in the morning, return home for a nap at two each afternoon, then go back to the office for the rest of the afternoon. J. R. R. Tolkien would likewise return home from lectures or tutorials for lunch and a nap, then go back to his office in the midafternoon. (The habit of going home for lunch was once fairly common, but as commutes have gotten longer, it has become harder to sustain.) Jonathan Franzen discovered napping when he was writing *The Corrections*. He had recently stopped smoking and so was deprived of his usual habit of taking a smoking break when his energy flagged; instead, he started taking "wonderful, intense" short naps. After twenty minutes, he would "come surging back up to the surface and go straight to the desk and write." They were "some of the best weeks of writing I'll ever have," he later said. It was "when I came into myself as a writer." Author Haruki Murakami takes power naps "a lot," he writes. "Usually I get sleepy right after lunch, plop down on the sofa, and doze off" for thirty minutes. "As soon as I wake up, my body isn't sluggish and my mind is totally clear." Science fiction writer William Gibson has a nap after lunch. "Naps are essential to my process," he says. He doesn't dream about his writing while napping, but he does appreciate "that state adjacent to sleep, the mind on waking." Having already completed his four hours of focused writing in the morning, Thomas Mann napped for an hour in the late afternoon before attending to letters or short essays. Stephen King divides his writing days up simply: write in the morning, devote the afternoon to "naps and letters," and have the evenings free.

Even people who were famous workaholics broke up their day with a nap. Brazilian architect Oscar Niemeyer, who in his nineties still spent ten hours a day in his Rio de Janeiro studio, lay down after lunch. Architects Frank Lloyd Wright and Louis Kahn, both famous for their obsessive work habits, would nap in the afternoon, lying down on hard surfaces so they wouldn't oversleep. Thomas Edison's long hours in the laboratory were celebrated (partly thanks to Edison's gift for self-promotion), but he also had a tremendous capacity to fall quickly into a deep, restorative sleep for an hour or two. Alfred Tate, his personal secretary, called the catnap Edison's "secret weapon" and declared, "His genius for sleep equaled his genius for invention." Henry Ford was surprised during a visit to Edison's lab to find that the inventor was unavailable because he was asleep. "I thought Mr. Edison didn't sleep much," Ford told Edison's assistant. "Oh, he doesn't," the assistant replied. "He just naps a lot."

For some people, an afternoon nap is a way to stretch out the working day. Churchill's habit of an afternoon nap and bath may seem fussy, but his valet, Frank Sawyers, observed, "The effect of this complete break is usually to make two working days out of one—and he literally does twice the amount of work of the average person and exerts himself for twice the length of the conventional eight-hour day." A long afternoon nap let Lyndon Johnson have a "two-shift day" as president: he could start the day at 6 a.m. and end it the next morning at 2 a.m. Frank Lloyd Wright likewise advised architecture students that in the afternoon "a short nap was a must," as it "divided one day into two and helped to refuel the creative spirit."

WHY DO NAPS do you good? The most obvious benefit of napping is that it increases alertness and decreases fatigue. A short nap of around twenty minutes boosts your ability to concentrate by giving your body a chance to restore depleted energy. But regular naps—the habit, not just a single nap—have other benefits.

Regular napping can improve memory. Just as the brain uses a good night's sleep to fix memories, so too does it use naps to consolidate things you've just learned. Neuroscientist Sara Mednick found that napping for an hour or more during the day—a nap long enough to allow one to dream—improves performance on memory and perceptual tasks. In a study published in 2003, she had people learn a texture discrimination task in the morning. If you've ever been to the eye doctor, you've probably had a peripheral vision test: you focus your attention on a light into the center of a large screen and push a button when when you see a light on the periphery. Mednick's test was a bit similar. Subjects were shown a field of little horizontal lines with an L or T in the center. After an irregular interval, some of the lines in the lower left morphed into diagonals. Subjects had to indicate when they saw the change, whether the lines formed a horizontal or vertical row, and what the central fixation target was (partly to keep people from just focusing on the lower left-hand quadrant). It's a simple test, but this sort of visual discrimination is the kind of thing our brains are designed for, and you can quickly get pretty good at it.

After the test, subjects were divided into three groups. One group didn't nap at all and went about their normal days. The other two took either an hour-long or ninety-minute nap in the afternoon. Everyone was then retested that evening. The subjects who didn't have a nap did worse on the test. Among the subjects who napped, though, Mednick found that a third had essentially the same scores, while two-thirds did dramatically better in the evening.

So a nap was helping the brain fix this new pattern-recognizing skill. But what accounted for the two sets of results among the nappers? It wasn't just the length of the nap: while the ninety-minute nappers were almost all in the high-performance group, people who slept an hour were split between both groups. Mednick found the answer when she looked at EEG tracings of their sleeping brains. When you sleep, you go through a 90-to-110-minute-long cycle that proceeds from light sleep to deep slow-wave sleep and finally to REM sleep. In REM sleep, your eyes twitch (REM stands for "rapid eye movement"), your brain waves pick up again, and you're more likely to dream. The balance of slow-wave and REM sleep varies depending on when you fall asleep and how tired you are. Some people had fallen into slow-wave sleep during their naps, while others had had both slow-wave *and* REM sleep. The slow-wave sleep group performed the same on the morning and evening tests. The slow-wave and REM sleep group, though, were the high performers. Finally, Mednick had the subjects take the same test again the next morning, and then two days later. Everyone's scores went up after a night's sleep, but the nap group's scores rose more sharply than the non-nap group.

Other researchers have found that even a short nap can improve memory. At the University of Düsseldorf, Olaf Lahl showed two groups of students a list of thirty words for two minutes and told them to memorize as many as possible. One group was then allowed to nap for up to an hour, while the other stayed awake. When they were tested to see how many words they could recall, the students who napped did significantly better than those who didn't. In a second experiment, one group was kept awake, a second napped as long as they wanted (about twenty-five minutes on average), and a third was woken up after five minutes. Lahl found that even a five-minute nap yielded measurable improvements in retention: not as great as a longer nap, but still statistically significant.

The effect isn't confined to humans: rats' cognitive abilities are also improved by naps, as a team at University College London led by neuroscientists Hugo Spiers and Freyja Ólafsdóttir discovered. They put electrodes in the brains of rats, then put the rats in a simple T-shaped track with food at the end of the short arm. As they ran up and down the long arm of the track, the rats could see the food and see how to get to it, but their path was blocked. When the rats rested, their brains' place cells, a set of specialized brain cells that store information about places you've visited and that are used when navigating, were especially active. The place cells that were associated with the arm that had food were lighting up; the cells that represented the empty arm, in contrast, were more dormant. Their brains appeared to be "playing out" the path to the food, solidifying this new information and imagining how to use it in the future.

Naps can also help workers avoid mistakes and bad behavior. Jennifer Goldschmied, a graduate student at the University of Michigan, found that naps improve emotional regulation and self-control. She measured her subjects' levels of tolerance for frustration by giving them paper, a pencil, and a set of diagrams. They had to copy the diagrams without lifting their pencil from the paper or tracing over a line. What they didn't know was that half the diagrams couldn't be copied without violating one of those rules. The participants thought they were being tested on their visual acuity or problem-solving skills, but Goldschmied really wanted to see how much time they would spend trying to come up with a solution before they quit. She found that people who had taken a nap before trying to complete the Frustration Tolerance Task were less likely to give up than those who hadn't napped, were less impulsive, and were better able to handle frustration. In separate studies, Dan Ariely and Christopher Barnes found that chronic fatigue or mental exhaustion decreases a person's self-control and decision-making ability, making them more likely to impulsively cheat than their better-rested colleagues.

Short twenty-minute power naps are good for boosting alertness and mental clarity. But sleep researcher Sara Mednick argues that by paying attention to what time of day you nap and scheduling longer naps with an eye to your sleep cycle and the highs and lows in your energy and attention levels (which follow an ultradian rhythm, rising and falling repeatedly through the day), you can tailor naps to be more physically restorative, to feed your creative activities, or to improve your memory.

Mednick did some of the first work that scientifically measured the benefits of naps. By the time she started graduate school at Harvard in the late 1990s, sleep scientists had developed a whole toolkit to study the effects of nocturnal sleep and sleep deprivation on things like memory, alertness, and perception. Mednick applied some of those tools to study naps. Previously, researchers had mainly been interested in naps in the context of shift work and sleep deficits; no one had paid much attention to how naps could affect the cognitive performance or alertness of people with stressful or challenging lives but more regular schedules. To her surprise, she found that a sixty- or ninety-minute nap provided the same kinds cognitive improvements seen in people who had slept for eight hours. (That's not to say you can trade a night's sleep for an afternoon nap. It doesn't work that way.) Further, she found that timing your nap can affect the balance of light sleep, REM sleep, and slow-wave sleep, and shape the kinds of benefits you get from it.

Sleep scientists have long observed that our need for sleep is governed by two things: sleep pressure and our body's twenty-four-hour circadian rhythm. Sleep pressure is the body's need for sleep, and, under normal circumstances, it's what's responsible for our feeling sleepy at night. When you wake up refreshed in the morning, your sleep pressure is at a minimum, and it builds up over the course of the day, until it reaches a peak the next night. Circadian rhythm regulates your alertness level. Under normal circumstances, you reach peak alertness around 8 a.m. and 8 p.m.; your alertness dips a little in the early afternoon, then rises through the rest of the day until late evening.

Circadian rhythm and the sleep pressure cycle operate independently of each other. Under normal circumstances the two are in sync: when we go to bed, our circadian cycle is at its lowest ebb and sleep pressure is high; when we wake up, our circadian cycle is revving up and our sleep pressure is low. But they can be thrown out of sync by jet lag, night shifts, or irregular work schedules.

The interaction of the two cycles helps determine what kind of sleep you get. When sleep pressure is high, your body demands more short-wave sleep. This is one reason why, when you go to bed at night, the first phase of your sleep tends to be dominated by deep, restorative short-wave sleep. As the night progresses, sleep pressure is eased and the need for short-wave sleep declines. In the middle of the night, your circadian cycle hits bottom and then starts to climb upward; as it does, you shift into REM sleep. By the time you wake up, your brain has been getting more active for a couple hours.

Mednick discovered that you can use knowledge of the relationship between sleep pressure, circadian rhythm, and sleep type to tailor a nap to your needs. About six hours after you wake up, your body's circadian rhythm starts to dip and you're likely to feel drowsy, especially if you've had a busy morning and lunch. A twenty-minute power nap at this point (say at 1:00 p.m.) is enough to give you a mental recharge without leaving you groggy: if you keep it short, you'll wake up fairly alert and can quickly get back to work. If you stretch it out to an hour, the balance between your circadian rhythm and sleep pressure will produce a nap that balances REM and short-wave sleep. If, on the other hand, you take a nap an hour earlier, five hours after waking, the balance will be different: more REM sleep, less slow-wave sleep. This kind of nap will deliver a little creative nudge: you're likely to dream and more likely to enroll your subconscious in whatever you were recently working on. If you wait until an hour later, seven hours after waking, your body needs more rest, and an hour-long nap will be richer in slow-wave sleep and more physically restorative than creatively stimulating.

These aren't dramatic differences: no nap will consist exclusively of one phase of sleep, and no single nap will magically turn you into Albert Einstein (who did nap regularly, it should be noted). And it's also important to remember that there's always a gap between laboratory studies of memory, cognition, and creativity, and real-world creativity and work. Few of us have jobs that require us only to memorize strings of numbers or remember pictures, or think up unusual uses for tape. But like Marily Oppezzo's work on walking and creativity, Sara Mednick's work on naps helps explain why, throughout history, so many dedicated, obsessed, competitive people have, in the middle of the day, stopped what they were doing and gone to sleep, and why they benefit from it. Whether they're politicians and poets, highly creative and productive people nap like farm laborers or mechanics: the favored time for a nap has been the hour after lunch, which, if you're on a normal sleep schedule, produces a nap balanced in REM and slow-wave sleep. Of course, any nap is going to provide benefits: creative work is both mentally and physically demanding, so a physically restorative nap is likely to be as useful as a creatively energizing nap. No sleep is going to be lost time.

WHILE LOTS OF active and creative people have discovered that naps help them recharge, a few use naps to generate insights. These people are much rarer, but it's worth looking at how they napped and what they claimed to get out of naps.

Edgar Allan Poe claimed that his literary experiments were enhanced by his ability to stay on the edge of a nap, to hold off "the lapse from this border-ground into the dominion of sleep," remaining in a state "when the bodily and mental health are in perfection" and "the confines of the waking world blend with those of the world of dreams." French poet André Breton traced the beginnings of his career as a surrealist to a breakthrough in 1919 when, "in complete solitude and at the approach of sleep," his mind began to form "sentences, more or less complete, which became perceptible to my mind without my being able to discover (even by meticulous analysis) any possible previous volitional effort." Science fiction writer William Gibson says, "Naps are essential to my process. Not dreams, but that state adjacent to sleep, the mind on waking." These writers all learn to linger in the hypnagogic state, the transitional phase between being awake and asleep.

But the most devoted and systematic user of naps to harvest creative ideas was Spanish painter Salvador Dalí, who describes his method in his 1948 book *Fifty Secrets of Magic Craftsmanship*. Much of Dalí's advice in the book is as . . . well, surreal as you would expect. Beethoven's practice of counting out exactly sixty beans for his morning cup of coffee has nothing on Dalí's instructions for getting inspiration from the eyeballs of sea perch cooked in fennel. And his observation that "a gradual pressure" exerted on the eyeballs "by an appropriate pneumatic apparatus, will make you dream in color" is slightly unsettling. Which makes it interesting that his advice about how to nap, and how to use naps to stimulate your creativity, is rather more practical. Dreams are a product of the roiling chaos of the subconscious, but Dalí finds they can be harnessed in a systematic way. Like other creatives, Dalí approaches inspiration in a surprisingly orderly way.

Dalí argues that the real work of painting happens while the artist sleeps, particularly in the nights before starting a new painting. He urges readers not to regard this sleep as a period of "inactivity and indifference." To the contrary: "It is precisely during this sleep," he says, "that you will secretly, in the very depths of your spirit, solve most of its subtle and complicated technical problems, which in your state of waking consciousness you would never be humanly capable of solving." It is in the dream that "the principal part—that is to say the sleep—of the work is already done." To use Graham Wallas's terms, the preparation and incubation phases happen while the artist prepares a work, doing preliminary sketches and staring at the canvas. The illumination happens as the artist dreams. But its products are locked in the artist's dreaming mind.

The key, then, is for the artist to learn how to access those insights as she works, to bring to the surface creative work that the subconscious has already done but that remain inaccessible to the everyday waking mind. The surrealists knew from Freud that one could develop techniques for recalling and accessing dreams, and they had a variety of techniques for tapping the unconscious. Dalí calls his technique for accessing dream imagery—the insights his unconscious had already produced, which only needed to be recovered—"slumber with a key."

The slumber itself is very short. "Your afternoon sleep must last less than a minute, less than a quarter of a minute," he advises, for two reasons. Long naps "'enslave' you by their heaviness for the whole rest of the afternoon," leaving you unable to work; manual laborers who engage in "violent physical exertions" can indulge in the traditional siesta, but the artist needs to avoid them. A very brief nap provides enough time for insights from the dream world to surface, but not enough time for you to forget them. By balancing "on the taut and invisible wire which separates sleeping from waking," you reach a state in which you can access both the creativity of the unconscious mind and conscious memory.

To do this, Dalí instructs readers to nap "in a bony armchair, preferably of Spanish style," with your hands over the side of the chair, palms facing up. Hold a heavy key between thumb and forefinger of the left hand. Then, "let yourself be progressively invaded by a serene afternoon sleep, like the spiritual drop of anisette of your soul rising in the cube of sugar of your body."

As you begin to drift off, your hand will relax, the key will fall, and the sound of it striking the floor—or, better yet, a metal plate on the floor—will wake you up in the seconds after some of the images from your dream appear. Instead of having to struggle to remember them, as we often do, you'll stay just conscious enough to remember them easily.

A few minutes in this state—almost falling asleep, startling awake, sketching or writing down the images that surfaced in the seconds before the key hit the floor, then settling back with the key in one hand—will be enough to tap the reservoir of insight, restore your energy (an important benefit for Dalí, who favored ample lunches and champagne), and guide your afternoon's work.

According to Dalí expert Bernard Ewell, Dalí would "float along" in this state for some time "while his imagination would churn out the images that we find so fascinating, evocative, and inexplicable when they appear in his work."

What's happening here? Psychologists call these moments between consciousness and sleep the hypnagogic sleep state (from the Greek *hupnos*, "sleep," and *agōgos*, "leading to"). It's like REM sleep, Montreal psychologist Michelle Carr explains: REM sleep and hypnagogia are both states in which "the mind is fluid and hyperassociative" and can more easily "bring together distant ideas in a new way." Inhibitions that keep your conscious mind from accessing unconscious processes and ideas are weakened. You haven't yet moved through the open gate between consciousness and unconsciousness. By staying just on the conscious side, you allow images from your subconscious to escape. In those few seconds before your hand drops the key, the mind enters a state that is "the essence of the dialectics of the dream," as Dalí puts it.

It's also important to note that the images that bubbled up from Dalí's subconscious were not completely spontaneous. Dalí's work is famous for its dreamlike, even hallucinatory quality. It's easy therefore to imagine Dalí rushing to the canvas to paint after a moment of sudden, unexpected inspiration, shocked into action by a vision. But that's not how it worked. Dalí used hypnagogia to access the inventory of images that his dreaming mind had generated while he was preparing his next work, thinking about solutions to the "subtle and complicated technical problems" presented by the next painting.

Edgar Allan Poe's use of hypnagogia wasn't the work of a dilettante, either. By the time he described his use of hypnagogia in 1845, Poe had spent half his life as a writer, poet, critic, and editor. André Breton's first encounter with creative hypnagogia came early in his career, but after working in the neurology ward of a hospital during World War I, applying Freudian practices to shell-shocked soldiers, and working on his poetry on the side, its appearance was far from random. For all three, hypnagogic imagery appears after a period of preparation, as Graham Wallas described.

The idea of using hypnagogic naps as a way of charting one's own subconscious and retrieving ideas generated in it is tantalizing. For those who want to try it but don't have an artist's studio, University of Montreal psychologist Tore Nielsen recommends a variation that can be done at one's desk. In his Upright Napping Procedure, when you start to feel drowsy, don't fight it; instead, close your eyes, relax, and let yourself drift toward sleep. With practice, the involuntary movements your body will make as you get drowsy can prevent you from nodding off for too long and wake you up in time to write down what came to mind as you were falling asleep.

It's a bit less eccentric than Dalí's method and better suited to an office: your coworkers might not appreciate the heavy sound of a falling object hitting the ground repeatedly. But as Dalí warns his readers, this is not something that comes naturally. "To achieve a painter's slumber," he warns, "will, in fact, require a long period of training." Dreams offer access to the unruly, creative depths of the unconscious, but dreaming—at least, dreaming like an artist—is a skill that takes time to learn.

IN MUCH OF the world today, naps have fallen out of favor. They're now something that young children do on kindergarten mats, not something for adults, least of all leaders and serious minds. As we move into a world and economy that seems to defy the constraints of geography and time, that operates globally and twenty-four/seven, we feel the need (or pressure) to work continuously, to ignore our own body's clocks and push on even when our bodies are pleading to rest. But this is a mistake. Naps are powerful tools for recovering our energy and focus. We can even learn to tailor them to give us more of a creative boost, or provide more physical benefit, or explore the ideas that emerge at the boundary between consciousness and sleep. Even during his country's most desperate hours, when he felt the fate of the nation and civilization hanging in the balance, Churchill found time for a nap. We would be wise to ask if our days and our work are really more urgent.

Stop

The best way is always to stop when you are going good and when you know what will happen next. If you do that every day . . . you will never be stuck. Always stop while you are going good and don't think about it or worry about it until you start to write the next day. That way your subconscious will work on it all the time. But if you think about it consciously or worry about it you will kill it and your brain will be tired before you start.

—Ernest Hemingway

A COUNTERINTUITIVE BUT EFFECTIVE form of deliberate rest is to stop working at just the right point: to see your next move, but leave it until tomorrow. Ernest Hemingway was a famous advocate of the practice, and many notable writers have followed his advice to "always stop when you know what is going to happen next." Stopping work on a project when you can see the next point to make, or when you still have a little energy left, makes it easier to get started the next day. It helps create a steadier pace that makes you more productive in the long run. It also seems to tease your subconscious mind into thinking about your work while you're doing other things.

"My rule is quit when I'm hot," said Allan Burns, the screenwriter whose credits included *The Munsters* and *The Mary Tyler Moore Show* (and who during his years in advertising created Cap'n Crunch). According to *Mad Men* showrunner Matthew Weiner, Burns would stop when he was "in the middle of something and it's good and [he knew] where it's going to go"; that way, "when [he got] back tomorrow [he could] get back on it." Many writers stop at that point so they can stay hot the next day. Roald Dahl was always careful to leave something unfinished so that he would "never come back to a blank page" in the morning, he said. Salman Rushdie said, "When I stop for the day I always try to have some notion of where I want to pick up" the next morning. Mario Vargas Llosa would "always leave a few lines untyped," making the next morning's first work "like a warm-up exercise." Even the Cambridge mathematician John Littlewood noted that while "the natural impulse towards the end of a day's work is to finish the immediate job," it was preferable to "try to end in the middle of something," since it was always easier to start the morning by going over "the latter part of the previous day's work."

The deliberate stop also makes you more productive over the long run. Many writers start their careers believing that the best work is done in bursts of inspiration only to discover that they do higher-quality work and get more done if they pace themselves. Early in his career, science fiction author Neal Stephenson believed that a good writer would write all day, but after losing a couple years to "a miserable, incoherent pile" of a book, he tried a more disciplined approach, learned to stop in mid-thought so that "the next morning there'd be something in the buffer, waiting to be written down," and quickly finished *Zodiac*. As a young writer, John McPhee would stay at the typewriter until the middle of the night, but gradually he realized that he paid for it the next day and his overall productivity suffered. "If I am in the middle of a sentence, and I'm all excited and it's really going well," he said, "I get up and go home." Getting a good pace and rhythm going when undertaking a complex project is as important for a writer as it is for a long-distance runner. Creative work is a marathon, not a sprint, as writer (and marathoner) Haruki Murakami put it. In both running and writing, "once you set the pace, the rest will follow," Murakami says. "The problem is getting the flywheel to spin at a set speed—and to get to that point takes as much concentration and effort as you can manage." As an author, the most reliable practice is to "stop every day right at the point where I feel I can write more. Do that, and the next day's work goes surprisingly smoothly." For Stephenson, McPhee, and Murakami, getting deeply immersed for long periods in their work is not a problem; the challenge is to turn that potentially destructive force into a sustainable source of creative energy.

Hemingway had one other reason for recommending that writers end the workday in mid-sentence. If you stop in the middle, he said, "your subconscious will work on it all the time. But if you think about it consciously or worry about it you will kill it and your brain will be tired before you start." Hemingway intuited that in the long run he would do better work if he gave his subconscious free rein and free time to work, and that his subconscious would do better work if he tempted it with an uncompleted idea. After he became a full-time writer, John le Carré would "go to sleep on a good idea and wake up with the idea solved or advanced," he said.

The discovery of the default mode network and mind-wandering suggests that Hemingway's intuition was correct and his subconscious carried on without him. Indeed, since Graham Wallas first argued for the importance of incubation in the creative process, psychologists have tried to understand why breaks help with insight. Whether they've looked at memories of creative people or measured the effects of breaks on performance on divergence tests, they've found that breaks provide a fairly consistent boost to creative thinking. For a long time, the why has been elusive. The two competing positions were nicely summarized by Henri Poincaré. "It might be said that the conscious work has been more fruitful because it has been interrupted and the rest has given back to the mind its force and freshness," he wrote. "But it is more probable that this rest has been filled out with unconscious work." Some psychologists, following Wallas, argued that the break gave the subconscious time to work. Others argued that a break simply provided a chance for the brain to recover some of the energy it had previously expended, just as a break lets athletes catch their breath. But studies of the brain's resting state and default mode network challenged the break-as-recovery model. Even when you're just staring into space, your brain uses only 5–10 percent less energy than it does when you're focused on a difficult task.

This suggests that the creative benefits of breaks are more likely to be the product of an active subconscious process. A group of researchers at the University of Sydney's Center for the Mind explored this question in a series of experiments. In one experiment, ninety students were asked to come up with as many novel uses as possible for a piece of paper. Some of them worked for four minutes without a break. Others worked for two minutes, then worked on a similar kind of test for five minutes, then (to their surprise) were asked to spend two more minutes thinking about paper uses. A final group worked for two minutes, did something completely different for five minutes, then spent two more minutes on the paper task.

All three groups came up with an average of fourteen responses in the first two minutes and fewer in the second two minutes. This is not surprising; what was interesting was that the first and second groups generated about seven responses in the second two minutes, but the third—the group that switched to a different task for five minutes—outperformed them both, generating almost ten ideas in the second two minutes. The experiment showed that having "a break during which one works on a completely different task is more beneficial for idea production than working on a similar task or generating ideas continuously." Divergence test scores rose not because people's brains had a chance to recharge but because their minds were able to switch to a different task. The results made the muscle theory look pretty iffy.

The researchers next asked, do highly creative people's brains benefit more from breaks than normal people's brains? If incubation is one of the critical points in the creative process, they reasoned, and breaks provide time for incubation, then creative people might get a bigger boost from breaks than everybody else. The subjects in their study first spent two minutes doing a divergent thinking task, then five minutes on math problems, then another two minutes on divergent thinking. This time, half the participants knew that they'd be tested twice; for the other half, the second test was a surprise. This let the researchers measure how awareness that you'll be returning to a problem affects how much your subconscious continues plugging away, looking for ever-more imaginative uses for a brick. (The math problems were difficult enough to keep participants' minds from consciously returning to the divergence test, and participants were told that their performance would be evaluated by how well they did on the math test, so they had an incentive to focus on them.)

When they analyzed the results, comparing the test scores before and after the break, they found that all scores went up on the second test. Everybody benefited from taking a short break. This was reassuring: they'd expected to see such a bump, as researchers had for decades. But they also found that people who went into the math break in the "aware condition," who had been warned that they'd be tested a second time, did far better on the second test than those in the "unaware condition," who didn't know that the experiment would continue after the break. Knowing that they were going to be tested a second time gave their subconscious minds a kick.

The research also revealed something even more interesting: people in the aware condition who came up with a larger number of creative responses got a bigger charge from the break than other subjects. In other words, their subconscious minds worked harder during the break than less-creative people. What this means is that "creative people are better able to utilize nonconscious processes" than the average person, and "the activation of such processes is greatest when a future task is anticipated."

The Sydney group's research suggests why Hemingway's method works and, more generally, why keeping to a schedule can clear the ground for the insight—why, as Picasso put it, inspiration must find you working. Stopping in midsentence makes it easier for you get back into the rhythm of your writing when you resume: having a couple of easy lines of dialogue to type, rather than starting with a new and unfamiliar scene, helped Hemingway get going in the morning. Having the sentence turning over in your mind puts you in the aware condition: you know you're going to go back the next day, finish that sentence, and keep going. And whether you know it or not, part of your mind is also writing the next sentence, and the next paragraph; considering and discarding a thousand plot twists without your ever being aware of them; and doing all kinds of other work. It would be doing that anyway; our brains are remembering, considering alternate paths, and thinking about the future all the time, and only sometimes are we aware of that (when we daydream, for example, or are trying to read a textbook and realize we're thinking about our last vacation). Creating an aware condition for yourself puts your brain on higher alert. We're going to take this up again in the morning, your mind says. Better keep going.

WRITER AND FORMER professional cricketer Ed Smith drew a parallel between his experience as a writer and his former career as an athlete. Smith reached the peak of his game when he practiced hard for four hours a day (broken into two two-hour sessions, like the schedules of the Berlin conservatory violinists) and was self-aware enough to know when to stop. As an athlete, he writes, "stopping practising at the right moment is a vital form of self-discipline, every bit as important as 'putting the hours in' and 'giving it your all.'" The same is true of creative work, he argues. We assume that constant, ceaseless effort yields high performance and that people who are constantly busy must be getting more done. Today's workplace respects overwork, even though it's counterproductive, and treats four-hour days as "contemptibly slack," even though they produce superior results.

But you don't do great work by sprinting to the finish; you're more likely to accomplish great things by stopping at a strategic point and continuing the next day. Learning to stop at the right point in your work encourages a steadier, more sustainable approach to your work, without sacrificing creativity or forcing you to extremes. Like designing a distraction-free morning, cultivating a routine that creates space for both focused work and fulsome rest, and using walks and naps to restore creative energy and promote creative insight, stopping at the right time requires understanding the demands of your work, learning to monitor your energy and attention, and appreciating how focused attention and mind-wandering can become partners in creative enterprises, and in a creative life.

Sleep

If sleep doesn't serve some vital function, it is the
biggest mistake evolution ever made.

—ALLAN RECHTSCHAFFEN

S LEEP IS THE original deliberate rest. For a long time, we
viewed sleep simply as a period in which we are inactive,
mind and body shut down. But since the 1930s, sleep scientists have put electrodes on the scalps of sleeping people,
measured their involuntary movements, even prevented them
from dreaming and measured the effects on their mental
state. What they've discovered is that sleep isn't the passive
phase we imagine (or experience) it to be. While you sleep,
your brain is busy consolidating memories, repairing physical
damage, and generating dreams. Most of the time you're not
aware of all this work, but it's been going on your whole life.
And your life depends on it. Sleep deprivation has immediate effects on your ability to focus, make good judgments,

perform under pressure, and be creative. Long-term sleep deprivation can affect your mental health and physical condition. Given how much humans sleep, it makes sense that evolution has packed lots of activities into those hours.

Sleep is an entirely natural activity—if you have a brain, at least. Plants and bacteria follow circadian rhythms, becoming more active at certain times of day and less at other. Even organisms that live less than twenty-four hours, like cyanobacteria, follow a fragment of a circadian rhythm. Plants in temperate climates become dormant in the winter to protect themselves from the cold and conserve energy. But plants and bacteria don't sleep. Insects sleep; indeed, some sleep researchers now study genetic mutations in *Drosophila melanogaster*, the fruit flies that have been a staple of genetics research for more than a century. (Keep in mind, though, that there are millions of species on Earth, and scientists have named only a minority of them—1.2 million of 8.7 million, according to a 2011 estimate—seriously studied a fraction of that minority, and studied the sleep patterns in only a tiny slice of that fraction.)

All mammals sleep, but with huge variations. Generally, carnivores sleep more than omnivores, and herbivores need even less sleep than omnivores. Among herbivores, sleep time varies with mass: elephants need about four hours a night, while armadillos sleep twenty hours a day. Sleep patterns also vary widely: rodents nap for short periods throughout the day and night while primates sleep for longer, unbroken periods. Sleep is important enough for some to have developed impressive strategies for doing so without endangering their well-being. Dolphins and whales, who live in the open ocean and must regularly surface to breathe, are unihemispheric sleepers: half of their brain sleeps while the other half remains awake, keeping the animal moving and able to respond to threats. (Fur seals are unihemispheric sleepers when they're in the water and bihemispheric sleepers on land.) Among primates, humans are actually on the low end of the sleep scale. Nocturnal primates sleep a lot more than humans: the three-striped night monkey (*Aotus trivirgatus*), for example, sleeps seventeen hours a day, more than twice as much as the average human. But macaques sleep between nine and fourteen hours, baboons nine to eleven hours, and chimpanzees about ten. Humans, in contrast, sleep about seven hours a night on average, but we sleep more soundly and effectively.

We experience a good night's sleep as a break from our active lives, a period when we disconnect from our normal reality. Paradoxically, it's restful because our brains aren't really shutting down. In fact, we often wake up most restored and get the most out of a night's sleep when, unknown to us, our brains have been at their busiest. During the day, our bodies are mainly occupied with the business of living, spending energy on motor activity and cognitive functions. When we fall asleep, our bodies shift into maintenance mode and devote themselves to storing energy, fixing or replacing damaged cells, and growing, while our brains clean out toxins, process the day's experiences, and sometimes work on problems that have been occupying our waking minds. This work isn't evenly distributed through the night but is concentrated in those periods when we sleep most deeply.

A night's sleep feels like a single unbroken period, but our brains actually move through five different stages as we sleep. Our brain waves vary as we move from stage 1, the first and lightest phase (it's the one you're in when you just drift off for a moment in a lecture), to stage 2. After about fifteen minutes, our brain waves shift: the small bursts of activity that characterize the first two stages (charmingly called spindles and spikes) are supplemented by lower-frequency delta waves that mark the arrival of stage 3 and the first deep sleep of the night. (Stanford sleep research pioneer William Dement, who spent decades looking at EEG waves, compares stage 1 and 2 waves to waves breaking on a beach and stage 3 to slower ocean swells.) A few minutes later, the stage 1 and 2 waves disappear completely, the delta waves deepen, and we drop into the deepest phase of sleep, stage 4 or slow-wave sleep. Finally, when we enter REM sleep, we move our limbs, toss and turn, and rapidly move our eyes. We're not aware of any of this movement, but it reflects a higher level of brain activity: most of our dreaming happens during REM sleep.

If our daily lives are defined by cycles of work and rest, and our lives are improved by hard work and deliberate rest, our best sleep is a blend of active REM sleep and more passive slow-wave sleep. It's in these stages that brain growth and repair, memory consolidation, and dreaming take place.

When we reach stage 4 sleep, our bodies release a growth hormone referred to by the acronym GHRH (for growth hormone–releasing hormone). GHRH helps bruises and cuts, and fights off infections at the cellular level. GHRH stimulates the repair of cells, the growth of replacement cells, and, in children and adolescents, the creation of the new cells their bodies need to grow. GHRH also induces sleepiness. One reason fast-growing teenagers need so much sleep is that their GHRH levels are higher than their parents' or grandparents', and in laboratory experiments GHRH has been shown to help people with sleep problems get a better night's rest. Conversely, a lack of sleep can inhibit cellular repair and growth. There's evidence that long-term sleep deprivation can stunt growth.

While the body grows thanks to GHRH generated during deep sleep, the brain itself becomes more complex thanks to biochemical processes that happen during REM sleep. Oligodendrocyte precursor cells (OPCs) generate myelin, a fat that covers and protects axons and is critical for proper neural function. (The production of myelin by OPCs in the brains of infants and children helps explain how they do smart things; the incomplete myelination of the prefrontal cortex in the brains of teens helps explain why they do stupid things.) When you're asleep, OPCs get busy producing myelin, and they are extra productive when the brain goes into REM sleep. OPCs produce other helpful chemicals when the brain is awake: as a University of Rochester Medical Center study led by Maiken Nedergaard puts it, it's beginning to look like our brains can either be "awake and aware, or asleep and cleaning up," but they can't do both at the same time.

Maiken Nedergaard's laboratory has investigated the role sleep plays in allowing the body to clear out toxins. Like the rest of the body, the brain produces waste products as it works. In 2013, Nedergaard's group explained just how the brains of mice deal with these toxins. The brain floats in a cushion of cerebrospinal fluid, just as the earth is largely covered by water. It's long been known that the fluid helps cushion the brain from shocks, and Nedergaard and her team reasoned that it could also serve other functions.

They first injected a tracking dye into the cerebrospinal fluid of mice and watched how much the fluid circulated when the mice were awake and when they were asleep. When the mice were awake, the fluid barely moved; once they fell asleep, though, the fluid got busy. They tracked it moving along the same channels in the brain that hold blood vessels (a bit like cables in a trench).

But why did the fluid start flowing when the mice fell asleep? When we think about the brain, we mainly imagine its neurons and synapses, the cells and connectors that are responsible for cognitive activity. But most of the brain actually consists of a different kind of cell: neuroglial cells, or glia. Traditionally these were assumed to act like scaffolding or insulation, holding neurons in place and protecting them from injury, but recently they've been shown to play a much more active role in managing the brain. (Nedergaard's lab is actually called the Division of Glial Disease and Therapeutics.) While the neurons and synapses are busy with memory and cognition, the glia are managing brain chemistry and nerve signal propagation, and covering axons in myelin, which helps speed electrical signaling. If the neurons and synapses are the brain's creative workers, the glia are the cool office with lots of whiteboards and a kitchenette in which energy drinks and protein bars seem to magically appear.

The glial cells also help repair brain injuries, as Nedergaard and her lab had previously discovered. One type of glia, the astrocytes, build up in damaged areas, directing blood and nutrients, clearing away debris, blocking bacteria, and stimulating the neurons to rebuild. The glia also go to work during sleep: when they measured the volume of glial cells in mice brains, Nedergaard's team found that the glia shrank, expanding the channels and giving the cerebrospinal fluid more room to flow. (What signals to the glia that it's time to get busy? Noradrenaline, a hormone that seems to promote alertness, is also known to swell the glymphatic system, the network of glial cells. As mice fall asleep, noradrenaline levels decline, which allows the glia to shrink.)

Finally, the team measured the glial cells' ability to remove beta-amyloid, a protein that is present in high concentrations in the brains of people suffering from Alzheimer's disease. In the early 1990s, Harvard Medical School neurologist Dennis Selkoe proposed that the buildup of beta-amyloid interferes with the brain's normal function and that, in the cautious language of science, "gradual accumulation of the amyloid-β protein (Aβ) in brain regions serving memory and cognition is a precipitant of the earliest symptoms of Alzheimer's disease." If this theory is correct—and while the presence of the protein is well-established, the precise details of how the buildup triggers the disease are not—therapies that help the body clear beta-amyloid could reduce the odds of developing Alzheimer's. When Nedergaard's team injected a traceable beta-amyloid into the brains of mice, they found that the brains of sleeping mice flushed out the toxin twice as rapidly as those of awake mice.

YOU CAN ALSO measure the importance of sleep by looking at the impact of sleep deprivation. The military has extensively studied the effects of sleep deprivation on situational awareness, decision-making, and the ability to understand and follow orders. Since ancient times, warriors have seen a willingness to forgo sleep and sacrifice comfort for one's mission and comrades as signs of manly fortitude and self-denial. In modern militaries, commanders have accepted that sleep deprivation, like casualties, is simply an unavoidable fact of life during war, but assumed that with a combination of training, discipline, and fighting spirit, as well as coffee or "go pills," soldiers could perform indefinitely on just a couple hours' sleep per day. But recent experience shows that, especially in today's crowded, high-tech, high-tempo battlefield, sleep is not a comfort. It's a necessity.

Sleep scientists were able to get an especially clear picture of the impacts of sleep deprivation on combat readiness during first days of Operation Iraqi Freedom in 2003. The start of the Iraq War let scientists observe an army in a combat environment, dealing with all the complexities of mounting a complex, modern military operation and exposed to the stresses of sleep deprivation, while suffering few casualties from an opposing army. During the first week of ground operations, many soldiers and marines got only a couple hours' sleep per day, and after a couple days the effects of fatigue were visible: Humvee and Bradley Fighting Vehicle drivers falling asleep on the road, air crews stressed from round-the-clock sorties, sentries fighting to stay awake as they guarded bases, radar operators and gunners struggling to sort out friendly forces from the enemy.

Aviators serving in Iraq and Afghanistan had similar problems. B-2 pilots based at Whiteman Air Force Base in Missouri spent thirty-six hours in the air during runs over Iraq and as much as forty-four hours when bombing Taliban caves and strongholds in Afghanistan. After completing their missions, the planes would turn south for Diego Garcia, an airbase in the Indian Ocean, where they would land, refuel, and head home—a return trip that took another thirty hours. In a 2004 survey of pilots and navigators at Randolph Air Force Base in Texas, Air Force F-15 weapons systems officer Mary Melfi found that sleep deprivation and unintentional sleep were "common in cockpits throughout the USAF," thanks to a combination of extended mission times, poor scheduling, and disruptions of circadian rhythms. Officers reported that fatigue had affected their situational awareness, slowed their reaction times, or led to procedural errors or forgetfulness. Many had nodded off in the air during night operations or on long uneventful flights, or fought off sleep near the end of long missions.

In fact, in the first week of the war, 64 percent of all fatalities suffered by US and British forces were due to accidents or friendly fire, and fatigue was a factor in many of those deaths. (During the Vietnam War, in contrast, 81 percent of deaths were in combat rather than from disease, accident, or some other cause; in the Korean War and World War II, the percentage of soldiers killed who died in combat were 91 percent and 72 percent, respectively.)

Another set of studies has measured the effects of shift work on the performance and cognitive ability of doctors and nurses. The downsides of night work are well-documented, but it would be overstating things to suggest that hospital staff turn into well-trained zombies at night. A 2014 study of Danish surgeons found that while night work affects their circadian rhythms, surgeons can develop strategies to compensate for sleep deficits: senior physicians, who've learned over time how to manage the challenges of shift work, do a better job of it than interns. A 2015 comparison of mortality rates in US hospitals of patients who underwent exploratory laparotomy—a procedure where doctors cut through the abdominal wall to reach the internal organs—during the day and at night found no significant difference. However, a laparotomy is a pretty safe and familiar procedure, the sort of thing a surgeon ought to be able to do reliably, and it's not clear from the study that complicated emergencies can be handled as well. But a 2008 study of anesthesiology interns and anesthetists in New Zealand found that after a couple weeks of having night shifts or on-call duties layered atop their regular duties, their performance on psychomotor vigilance tests dropped. Not only that, a sleep deficit of less than an hour a night led to declines greater than those seen in comparable groups tested in a sleep lab. This suggests that laboratory studies might be underestimating the impact of sleep loss and that in the real world, the added stresses of making decisions, picking up kids, and trying to lead a normal life amplify the effects of sleep loss. Likewise, studies of night nurses in Saudi Arabia, Taiwan, and the United States all found that as their sleep quality declined, stress levels went up and cognitive performance dropped.

Sleep deprivation doesn't just erode your reflexes, decision-making, and ability to learn; it also has physical effects. Sleep deprivation lowers your immunity and erodes your body's ability to fight off infection. Night shift work throws off your sleep patterns and body clock enough to cause sleep deprivation. The normal cues your body uses to regulate its circadian rhythms—things like sunlight or darkness, warmth or cold—get thrown off when you sleep during the day and spend the night exposed to artificial light. Shift workers are more likely to develop ulcers, cardiovascular disease, and breast cancer. Even people who work night shifts for months or years on end tend to sleep less—about an hour less per night—and over the long run have higher rates of hypertension, obesity, diabetes, and other diseases.

Scientists are also seeing a connection between sleep deprivation and dementia. REM sleep behavior disorder (RSD), in which sleepers act out their dreams (sometimes even damaging nearby belongings, injuring themselves, or attacking spouses—RSD dreams tend to be violent), can be a precursor to hallucinations and dementia in people with Parkinson's disease, multiple system atrophy, or dementia with Lewy bodies. There's a high correlation between sleep disturbance and cognitive and functional impairment among people with Alzheimer's: people in the early stages of the disease sleep fairly normally, but as the disease progresses and memory and other cognitive functions decline, they become more likely to wake up in the middle of night and spend less time in deep stage 4 and REM sleep. It's not entirely clear whether the advance of dementia is accelerated by a decline in sleep quality, whether dementia erodes our ability to sleep well, or whether they share an underlying cause, but sleep researchers think that improving sleep at least slows cognitive decline, and there's some evidence that sleeping well in middle age provides some insurance against dementia later in life. Of course, bad sleep affects cognitive ability at any age, but the correlation between interrupted or abnormal REM sleep and dementia is another indicator that healthy brains use REM sleep to do work that keeps the brain in good shape.

Studies documenting the costs of sleep deprivation have led even notoriously hard-charging organizations to experiment with ways to help workers rest more and avoid the worst effects of sleep deficits. For shift workers, studies find that planned naps help alleviate (but, alas, do not eliminate) some of the problems inherent in shift work and night work. For example, a 2006 study of Brazilian nurses working nights in a hospital found that being able to nap during their shifts helped them deal with the stresses of working all night (particularly if they were working second jobs, which is pretty common) and improved their after-work recovery (that is, their ability to rest and mentally disengage from the job).

Likewise, the US military is starting to recognize that sleep deprivation isn't simply something to be overcome by sheer force of will and is slowly accepting that "strategic naps" are an effective way of dealing with fatigue. (Of course they have to be "strategic," to set them apart from the kind a three-year-old takes on a little mat at preschool.) A "prophylactic" nap taken before a night operation can be as useful as "repeated dosing of 150 mg of caffeine" (or, in civilian terms, drinking twelve-ounce cups of coffee). An "operational" nap taken during a mission can temporarily restore cognitive abilities and reflexes. Generally, naps taken later in a flight are more restorative than those taken earlier, as long as they're not taken so late that sleep inertia (the slowness you sometimes feel after waking up) threatens performance during landing. The number of hours you've been awake can also influence how restful a nap is and how long it takes to shake off any postnap grogginess.

A nap taken in a bunk or upright in the cockpit isn't going to replace a good night's sleep, but even a short nap can be surprisingly restorative. In the early 1990s, Mark Rosekind, a scientist at NASA's Ames Research Center in Silicon Valley, studied the effects of strategic napping on 747 crews flying across the Pacific. Transpacific flights are among the longest that civilian pilots fly: nonstop flights from San Francisco to Tokyo take eleven hours, while nonstop from Los Angeles to Hong Kong or Sydney takes fifteen. To make matters worse, half the flights leave the West Coast between midnight and 2 a.m., so if they've adjusted to California time, those crews have to wake up late in the evening, work through the night, and land planes the next morning after being awake for eighteen hours. When they touch down, their circadian rhythms think it's dinnertime, which makes it harder to get a decent interval of sleep before their next flight.

Rosekind wanted to know what effect strategic napping would have on crew alertness and performance, so he had one group of pilots power through the night while the other had a forty-minute window to nap. Both groups were evaluated on takeoff, vigilance, and landing. He found that the group that didn't rest had "reduced performance on night flights compared to days, at the end of flights compared to the beginning, and after multiple-flight legs." The group that was able to rest, in contrast, performed more consistently throughout the flight and on day and night flights.

Most impressive was the difference in the groups' performance during approach and landing. This is the most technically challenging and dangerous part of a flight. The flight crew has to put down the landing gear, slow the aircraft, and get into the proper flight path. At the same time they have to be aware of environmental conditions—turbulence, updrafts and downdrafts, rain or snow—and how they'll affect the final approach. They also have to pay closer attention to their surroundings—the sky around an airport is a lot more crowded than the sky at thirty-five thousand feet. And they have to do it all when they're most likely to be tired and jet-lagged. The NASA researchers observed 120 incidents of what they called "micro-events associated with physiological sleepiness" among the crews that hadn't slept: in other words, as they were heading into final approach, putting down the landing gear, deploying flaps to slow the plane (but not too much), communicating with air traffic control, and so on, the crews were fighting to stay awake: on average, their bodies started to fall asleep twenty-two times during approach and landing. The group that napped, in contrast, stayed wide awake.

So if you're fitter and frostier than fighter pilots and astronauts, forget about a nap. You don't need it. Otherwise, it's probably worth working a nap into your routine.

SLEEP GIVES THE brain a chance to repair itself; it also takes the time to process the day's events and solidify its memory of new skills. As we sleep, the brain shuffles around the day's memories, moving some from short-term to long-term memory. Visual tasks, emotionally laden experiences, and procedural memories (for example, hard-to-describe skills like riding a bike) tend to be consolidated during REM sleep, while declarative memories (things like lists of words) are consolidated during slow-wave sleep.

In the early 1990s, Israeli researchers tested the importance of REM sleep on memory. They taught two groups of people a visual discrimination task. They then allowed the groups to sleep and measured their performance on the test again the next day. Over the course of several nights, the researchers varied how the subjects slept: on some nights they were woken up whenever they started to enter REM sleep; on others they were left alone. They found that on days after they had slept normally, the groups' performance on the task improved; when their REM sleep was interrupted, however, their performance did not. Other experiments have found that people suffering from insomnia have impaired memory consolidation.

We also dream. Some of our most memorable dreams are vivid and surreal, but most seem to be more down-to-earth and involve replaying past events or reviewing problems. Neuroscientist Kieran Fox argues that "dreaming can be understood as an 'intensified' version of waking mind-wandering": the subjective experiences are similar, and some of the same regions of the brain are active during both dreaming and mind-wandering. The fact that we engage in task consolidation and performance review while sleeping might help explain why some people are able to dream about tasks. However, while stories like Friedrich August Kekulé's dream in which dancing snakes revealed the structure of the chemical compound benzene, or Samuel Taylor Coleridge's dreaming the poem "Kubla Khan," or Paul McCartney's dreaming the song "Yesterday" are examples of complete solutions revealing themselves in dreams, for most scientists, writers, and artists, sleep and dreams play a more indirect role in their creative lives. For example, at the end of the day, theoretical physicist Hans Bethe would talk with collaborators about the next day's work as a way of priming his sleeping mind. Linus Pauling made the practice of "thinking about certain scientific problems as [he] lay in bed, waiting to go to sleep" part of his problem-solving process. It might take weeks or months, but eventually the solution "would burst into [his] consciousness." The chemist Glenn Seaborg, who discovered ten new elements, would go to bed thinking about a problem and often "wake up at night or in the morning with a clear thought, a clear objective, a new idea." For Bethe, Pauling, and Seaborg, the answers to problems did not necessarily appear in dreams, but sleep and dreaming did help loosen ideas that became accessible during the waking day. Even athletes report harnessing dreams to help with problems they're working on: golf legends Ben Hogan and Jack Nicklaus both described dreams that helped them improve their golf swings.

Whether sleep generates a revelatory dream or helps accelerate problem-solving, these insights don't come out of nowhere. Instead, they follow Graham Wallas's four-stage model of innovation, in which a period of preparation and an incubation phase consisting of a night or more of sleep precede a clarifying dream or morning epiphany.

It's also noteworthy that while figures like Pauling respect the mind's ability to continue working while they are asleep, they don't expect revelations in their sleep. Rather, they see their sleeping minds and waking minds as partners and recognize that each has abilities that complement the other. They treat sleep as active rest.

IN 1906, AMERICAN experimental psychologist Joseph Jastrow noted in his book *The Subconscious* that "the idler moments of contemplative revery are as essential to fruitful production as the intent periods of executive effort; the trough of the wave is as intrinsic a part of its progressive character as the crest." The work of sleep researchers and neuroscientists confirms Jastrow's century-old observation. Sleep turns out to be important for the maintenance of the brain's physical health and the growth of new brain cells. It's essential for the consolidation of memories and processing of new skills, and for the interpretation of experiences. It even sometimes provides new insights and plays a role in maintaining a state of concentration, or "cerebral polarization," as Santiago Ramón y Cajal calls it.

More broadly, the unique properties of human sleep may have helped give rise to human society, intelligence, and culture. Primatologists have long noted that humans sleep less than other primates, and more recently sleep lab studies have revealed that other primates have shorter periods of slow-wave and REM sleep (the kinds that are especially important for memory consolidation and dreaming). Evolutionary biologists David Samson and Charles Nunn argue that short, deep sleep has played an important role in making humans smarter and more social. Shorter sleep left early humans less exposed to nocturnal dangers and predators and allowed them to use more of the day to gather food, care for young, develop new skills, and share knowledge with family and kin. Longer periods of slow-wave and REM sleep, meanwhile, helped humans get more out of each night's sleep. Seven hours of human-style sleep was enough to consolidate memories, restore the body, repair damaged cells, and clear out brain toxins. Together, longer waking days and nights of deeper sleep supported the growth of "enhanced cognitive abilities in early humans," while the need to sleep safely drove humans to adopt innovations like beds, shelters, controlled fires, and larger social groups.

So not only does sleep help us stay healthy, make sense of experiences, solidify memories, and generate new ideas, our species has been shaped by its unique sleep patterns. The partnership of waking and sleeping hours heightens our ability to learn and perform, while the character of our sleep deepens our ability remember and create, as individuals and as a species.

PART II

Sustaining Creativity

The best rest for doing one thing is doing another until you fall into a sound sleep. It is the vigorous use of idle time that will broaden your education, make you a more efficient specialist, a happier man, a more useful citizen. It will help you to understand the rest of the world and make you more resourceful.

—WILDER PENFIELD,
"THE USE OF IDLENESS"

Recovery

The supreme quality of great men is the power of
resting. Anxiety, restlessness, fretting are marks of
weakness.

—J. R. Seeley

In June 1942, Dwight Eisenhower was appointed Commanding General of the European Theater of Operations
for the US Army. Eisenhower was a well-respected thinker
and had risen rapidly through the army's senior ranks in
1940 and 1941, and his new position required overseeing
planning for the army's invasion of North Africa, working
with his British military counterparts, and fielding Winston
Churchill's demands for faster American action. When he
arrived in London, the war in Europe had already been going
on for nearly two years, and Eisenhower found a command
badly in need of reorganization and rejuvenation. By early
August, according to his aide Harry Butcher, Eisenhower

was working "15 to 18 hours a day" and had become a man "whose problems frequently [kept] him awake at night." Eisenhower ordered Butcher to find "a 'hideout' to escape the four forbidding walls of the Dorchester," the London hotel where the two shared a suite of rooms.

After scouting locations around London, Butcher found Telegraph Cottage, a "small, unpretentious" house "remotely situated on a 10-acre wooded tract." That summer and fall, while planning Operation Torch, the US invasion of North Africa, Eisenhower would escape to Telegraph Cottage whenever he could. There he played golf, read cowboy novels, played bridge, went riding in nearby Richmond Park, and simply enjoyed the country. An aide cooked simple American-style meals, a welcome change from formal British dinners. Shop talk was strictly forbidden. Only a handful of people outside Eisenhower's staff knew the cottage's location or ever visited. "If anything saved him from a mental crack-up," his driver, Kay Summersby, later said, "it was Telegraph Cottage and the new life it provided."

This kind of break from work—the kind that allows what sociologists call detachment, the ability to put work completely out of your mind and attend to other things—turns out to be tremendously important as a source of mental and physical recovery from work. It's essential for those in unpredictable, high-stress jobs that require lots of focus and emotional control, like nursing or law enforcement. It's equally essential for people who love their jobs, who are perfectionists and passionate. It's a necessity for people who want to do their very best work to be able to detach from the workplace, to have time to recover their mental and physical energy. For individuals, burnout can lead to emotional exhaustion, a decline in performance, poorer decision-making, lower empathy, and higher rates of errors. For organizations, burnout contributes to declines in productivity, a more stressed and unhappy workplace, and greater turnover. And it's often an organization's most talented and valuable workers who are most likely to burn out.

Dwight Eisenhower would go on to become one of the great heroes of World War II, celebrated as a brilliant general and a model of American confidence and character; but in 1942 he was a career staff officer thrown into his first major command and tasked with an immensely difficult high-stakes job. It was an early sign of his fitness for leadership that he recognized the need to restore his psychological reserves, to literally make space for rest. Eisenhower's hideout highlights the need to be able to detach from challenging and creatively demanding jobs to recover your energy and enthusiasm.

EXPERT OPINION ABOUT the best treatment for fatigue and exhaustion has generally fallen into two camps. In the nineteenth century, some doctors advocated a medically supervised "rest cure" for nervous exhaustion consisting of several bedridden weeks (sometimes in darkened rooms) and a bland diet; others argued that the tonic of fresh air, vigorous exercise, and primitive living was the best cure for nervous exhaustion brought on by the stresses of modern industrial civilization. (Not surprisingly, the former tended to be recommended for women and the latter for men.) In modern America, we tend to assume that the best way to recover our energy is to take a long leisurely vacation—that we have a reservoir of mental energy that we consume at work and time away from the office refills it. In this theory, the longer our vacations, the better.

This is one reason we've tended to take long vacations and spend generously on them. (The average American spent $4,580 on a family vacation in 2013, and well-heeled travelers spent an average of $13,000 on leisure travel in 2015.) But it's also one reason we don't take vacations: for many people, the idea of leaving the office for two or three weeks feels impossible, and the thought of facing a mountain of work and an overflowing inbox on their return is more stressful than never leaving. And the problem is getting worse: according to the US Travel Association, workers in 2000 took an average of twenty-one vacation days, but in 2013 that figure dropped to sixteen days.

But there are real costs to not taking vacations, too. American workers lose roughly $52.4 billion in earned benefits each year. They also lose long-term health benefits. The Framingham Heart Study found that over a twenty-year period, women who took infrequent vacations were more likely to have heart attacks than those who vacationed regularly. In a nine-year study of twelve thousand men at high risk for coronary heart disease, researchers found that those who took annual vacations had fewer heart attacks and lower overall mortality rates than men who did not. A 2015 survey found that 71 percent of workers who take regular vacations reported being satisfied with their work, versus 17 percent of workers who don't.

Workers who skip vacations or don't use all their vacation days cost their companies too. Unused vacation time weighs down company balance sheets to the tune of $224 billion, according to a 2015 study by Oxford Economics. Even more important, they're at higher risk of burnout, of feeling emotionally exhausted by their work and never feeling fully able to handle the demands of the job. Workers suffering from burnout become detached from work, are less empathetic to colleagues and customers, and feel that their work has little value, to themselves or the world; it can also create marriage and family problems and contribute to depression, poor health, and—especially among formerly hard-charging and career-oriented people—higher rates of suicide.

The effects of burnout in high-stress professions that require emotional balance and good judgment have been studied extensively. Law enforcement officers who suffer burnout are quicker to anger and to respond to difficult situations aggressively, and more likely to make mistakes. This is bad for policing, and for police: one study suggests that more officers are killed by job-related stress than die in the line of duty. Mayo Clinic physician Tait Shanafelt, who has been measuring the extent and impact of burnout on American doctors, found in surveys conducted in 2008 and 2010 that 40 percent of surgeons reported feeling burned out, 30 percent were depressed, and those who felt burned out were more likely to have made a "major medical error" in the previous three months. The Duke Divinity School's Clergy Health

Initiative found in a 2014 survey that 25 percent of full-time Methodist clergy suffered from emotional exhaustion, depersonalization, and a reduced sense of accomplishment (the three major symptoms of burnout), leading to poorer health and higher-than-average rates of obesity, hypertension, depression, and anxiety. (In fact, the term *workaholic* was first coined in a study of ministers.)

All this suggests that whatever short-term benefits come from overwork and delayed vacations, they're more than offset by the long-term costs of errors, lost productivity, higher turnover, and abbreviated careers. Exhausted workers can't give their best, take less initiative, are more cynical, and may even be actively subversive. Burnout is also most likely to affect the people employers can least afford to lose: their most dedicated, most experienced, and most skilled workers.

For writers, scientists, and entrepreneurs, delaying vacations can also mean passing up opportunities for creative breakthroughs. Lin-Manuel Miranda had the idea for *Hamilton* when he read Ron Chernow's biography of Alexander Hamilton during a vacation to Mexico. He had been working for seven years on his play *In the Heights,* and as he later put it, "the moment my brain got a moment's rest, *Hamilton* walked into it." Princeton physicist Lyman Spitzer came up with the design for a fusion reactor while skiing in Aspen, Colorado, in 1951. Software developers have epiphanies on vacation, too: Kevin Systrom came up with the idea for Instagram while on a vacation in Mexico in 2010, while Rafa Soto dreamed up OmmWriter, a minimalist word processor, on a beach in Brazil. In fact, according to a 2014 survey, one in five start-up founders got the idea for their company during vacations.

Given the high costs of exhaustion and burnout, it's worth asking what kinds of breaks provide the greatest degree of recovery. For the last twenty years, German sociologist Sabine Sonnentag has been exploring this question. Sonnentag's work assumes that emotional resources are as important for workers as physical energy is for athletes: however much you love the game, at some point you need to stop playing and rest. Along with a large number of collaborators (many of them graduate students who've gone on to distinguished careers of their own), she's studied how opportunities for recovery—the process of recharging the physical and emotional batteries— affect workers' health and well-being, job satisfaction, productivity, and resilience. She and her colleagues have looked at paramedics, clerical workers, software developers, civil servants, factory workers, consultants, schoolteachers, and the self-employed. She's measured the effects of time off and detachment on performance on multiple scales: the effect of weekends on energy levels during the week, of vacations on mood and work satisfaction months later, even the effects of being well-rested on energy and focus in the morning versus the afternoon.

Over the course of decades, across professions, in one industry after another, Sonnentag's findings have been consistent. Workers who have the chance to get away mentally, switch off, and devote their energies elsewhere, are more productive, have better attitudes, get along better with their colleagues, and are better able to deal with challenges at work.

They're also better able to focus intensely on work tasks. In one study, Sonnentag and her colleagues surveyed 120 software engineers and Web designers about the relationship between the quality of their nonwork time, how much they were able to recover in their off hours, and how often they got into highly focused flow states at work. The researchers expected to see a U-shaped pattern that followed circadian rhythms: a peak in the morning and later afternoon, when energy levels were high and sleep pressure low, with a midday trough when energy dips and sleep pressure increases. The well-rested programmers indeed experienced a drop in flow after lunch. Less well-rested programmers, in contrast, didn't follow the same pattern: their flow levels started low and steadily got worse.

Sonnentag and her colleagues argue that there are four major factors that contribute to recovery: relaxation, control, mastery experiences, and mental detachment from work. Think of them as a bit like vitamins. Breaks that are high in all four are the equivalent of nutritious and nourishing meals; those that don't are like empty calories.

Relaxation is the most straightforward of the four to understand: it's an activity that's pleasant and undemanding, or, as Sonnentag and her collaborator Charlotte Fritz define it, "a state of low activation and increased positive affect." By this definition, relaxation doesn't have to be totally passive: it just shouldn't feel like work or require conscious effort.

Control and mastery experiences are more interesting. In the context of recovery, control means having the power to decide how you spend your time, energy, and attention. For people who don't have much control over what happens at work and whose schedules are filled with family duties and chores, being able to control their time is liberating and re-storative. In a study of physicians and nurses in German hospital and psychiatric facilities, Sonnentag found that workers with more control over their time and attention felt less need to recharge at the end of the day; in contrast, workers with little control had more stress, worked longer hours, had less control over their daily routines or priorities, and had a greater need for recovery.

Mastery experiences are engaging, interesting things that you do well. They're often challenging, but this makes them mentally absorbing and all the more rewarding when you do them well. (These don't just make your vacation better, they make your life more meaningful: psychologist Mihaly Csikszentmihalyi has found that people who seek out flow experiences in difficult but rewarding activities are happier and have more satisfying lives than people who pursue sybaritic pleasures.) For people working in highly uncertain jobs, having mastery experiences during breaks can be especially important. In Bletchley Park during World War II, for example, chess was a popular pastime among code-breakers. The heads of the Enigma section had played on the British national chess team and recruited players on the belief that the game built the mental skills necessary to do cryptanalysis; yet playing the game remained a recovery experience. It was effortlessly absorbing and thus relaxing. A number of code-breakers were highly rated chess players, and the games gave them an opportunity to exercise mastery. Finally, it was

unambiguous and certain: the board, rules, moves, and op-
ponent were all in the open, unlike the murky world of codes
and ciphers.

The importance of psychological detachment as a factor in
recovery was first observed in a 1998 study by Israeli sociologists Dalia Etzion, Dov Eden, and Yael Lapidot of workers
before and after their annual service in the Israeli military.
Most Israeli adults serve in the military full-time after finishing high school and then continue as reservists, serving a few
weeks each year. Lapidot surveyed returning reservists about
their levels of engagement and energy on the job and found
that they reported significantly lower rates of job stress and
burnout than before their deployments; in fact, their results
looked just like those of people who had been on vacation.

This seems counterintuitive, but researchers in other countries have observed the same phenomenon. US Air Force
surveys found a similar effect among airmen after overseas
deployments: even when they're stressful, short deployments
can provide a respite from the usual routines of base life. (Of
course, unexpected or repeated deployments and long tours
that put stress on family and home life, erase those benefits.)
In 2011, a study of Canadian army reservists found that de-
ployment promoted recovery. Even though it can be physically and mentally challenging, reserve service provided a
respite from the stresses of civilian jobs.

So detachment—the ability to feel disconnected from the
job—turns out to be important in determining how much
you recover during breaks. This turns out to be as true for
evenings and weekends as long vacations.

Etzion then looked at business travelers. She surveyed employees at a high-tech company before, during, and after business trips, and found that levels of job stress and burnout dropped significantly after a trip. The effect was even more dramatic among women, for whom a business trip meant a break from household chores and childcare. Subsequent studies have found recovery effects even for people who travel for a living. A study by Sonnentag and Eva Natter of German flight attendants (whose work is both physically taxing and emotionally demanding) likewise found that they experienced greater recovery from work when staying in a hotel than when returning home. In a study of commercial pilots, Macquarie University psychologist Ben Searle found that pilots' detachment from work increased—but only when they stayed at hotels farther away from the airport.

Relaxation, control, mastery experiences, and detachment all work together to promote recovery. An activity that is challenging and absorbing, and pushes thoughts of work out of your mind, increases your sense of detachment. This helps explain why many noted scientists have been avid musicians. In the twentieth century, the cultured physicist-musician was a virtual stereotype: get four physicists in a room, one joke went, and you'd have a string quartet. These days, they're more likely to be a heavy metal band, like the one organic chemist and MacArthur fellow Carolyn Bertozzi played in during college with future Rage Against the Machine and Audioslave cofounder Tom Morello. Theoretical physicist and author Brian Cox was keyboardist for the pop group D:Ream while in graduate school; Brian May, lead guitarist for Queen, took time off from Imperial College London's astrophysics graduate program to play music. (He finally completed his dissertation in 2007.) Computer scientist and classically trained baritone Ben Kazez explains that there are similarities between working on software and music. "If I'm working on a piece of music I love, I have lots of ideas" about how to interpret it, he says, and "it's the same with apps." (His iPhone app Flight Track helped launch the market for real-time flight information.) A musical performance and a start-up both involve getting very talented people to work together and do great work on a deadline. You might think that their similarity would make music less useful as a form of recovery, but because doing it well demands commitment, concentration, organizational skill, and cooperation, and channels some of the same energy and skill normally used on the job into a completely different context, playing music serves to promote recovery from work.

Detachment also requires being able to escape work-related interruptions. Knowing that you've left your pager in your desk or are out of cell phone range makes it easier to relax or focus on your swing. This is one reason workers who carry work smartphones or other devices during non-work hours, or who have to keep in touch with the office while they're on vacation, have higher levels of stress and work-family conflict. But it's also critical to able to disconnect from work psychologically. A study of the cortisol levels of on-call workers found a negligible difference between their stress and alertness levels when they were at work and on call. Likewise, people who worry about work in their off hours have lower recovery rates than those who do not. At the end of a long week, you're more likely to be emotionally spent, which makes you more likely to dwell on negative things, or to just keep thinking about that upcoming project or the work that was pushed aside in order to deal with an emergency. It's harder to detach from work after long, demanding days, and being exhausted and cranky leaves you with less energy to switch mental gears—precisely when it's most essential to do so.

In their study of Israeli reservists, Etzion, Eden, and Lapidot noticed something else about the boost in happiness reported by reservists when they came back to work: after a month, the effect faded, and they were as happy (or as miserable) as they had been before they left. Psychologists have since discovered that a similar effect holds for even relaxing vacations: the benefits don't last very long. When they measure mood, energy levels, engagement, and happiness levels among workers before and immediately after a vacation, then weeks or months later, psychologists find that the emotional boost that a vacation provides lasts about three or four weeks. After that, your happiness and job satisfaction levels return to their prevacation levels: it's "lots of fun, quickly gone," as one article puts it. (And for perfectionists and workaholics, the fade-out effects happen even faster.)

This led to another question: at what point during vacation does happiness peak? When psychologists ask people how they feel during a holiday, they find that happiness levels rise rapidly during the first few days, peak around day eight, then either plateau or slowly decline. We think of the big annual vacation as a great way to recover from the stresses of a job, and while long vacations have their virtues—they let you travel farther and spend more time learning about local cultures, for example—long vacations don't translate into greater happiness.

These results further undermine the idea that our mental energies refill with time, rather than through activities that promote recovery. They also suggest that we should reassess the role of breaks, and the rhythm of vacations, in our lives. Regularly and decisively breaking from our jobs, disconnecting from the office in the evenings and on weekends, and choosing to do things that are relaxing, mentally absorbing, and physically challenging—in other words, engaging in a form of active rest—will promote recovery of our mental resources and make us more effective, productive, and focused. Rather than treating vacations as big, annual events that are completely separate from our working lives, taking shorter but more frequent vacations every few months provides greater levels of recovery. As Jessica de Bloom, a psychologist at the University of Tampere and vacation researcher, puts it, vacations are like sleep: you need to take them regularly to benefit.

EISENHOWER'S TIME AT Telegraph Cottage serves as a model of recovery theory, which explains why it was so valuable in helping him recover from the pressures of his first command. It was a space where Eisenhower could exercise mastery in long bridge games (a game he played brilliantly) or relax over novels and golf ("Ike's [golf] score is a military secret," Butcher joked, suggesting that for Eisenhower, golf was more relaxation than mastery). Cottage life also gave him a chance to exercise a rare level of control over his time (he sometimes took over the kitchen to cook his own breakfast, though his aide drew the line at letting the boss do the dishes).

More important, its location helped Eisenhower recover from work. Except for the "bomb holes on the golf course" adjacent to the cottage, Butcher said, it was "so peaceful you'd never know there [was] a war." When he arrived to take up his new post, Eisenhower quickly discovered that the Dorchester Hotel offered no escape from work: a number of senior ministers and British military leaders were living in the hotel, thanks in part to its modern construction and reputation as bombproof and fireproof. In contrast, Telegraph Cottage was private, and Eisenhower and his staff worked to make sure it remained so. Eisenhower kept its location a secret from all but his closest aides. He didn't entertain guests or make deals over rounds of golf on the nearby course. He didn't bring work there, and Butcher and Bedell Smith avoided shop talk. Aside from his dog (who, revealingly, was named Telek, an abbreviation of "Telegraph Cottage"), the cottage and the life he maintained there was Eisenhower's great respite from the war, a key to staying sharp and recovering from the pressures of the job.

The story of Telegraph Cottage should remind us that even people in very high-stakes jobs need to set aside time for recovery. It's easy to forget that we need to build rest into our schedule. It's easy to convince ourselves that detaching from work is impossible. We live in an era when we're urged to be passionate about our work, to regard the boundary between work and life as an obsolete relic of the industrial age. Mobile technologies keep us connected to the workplace day and night. At the same time, the boundaries between work and life are blurred, giving us more flexibility and choice about how to organize our time. Together, they create the illusion that we'll find greatest fulfillment, and be most effective, if we're always working.

But that's wrong. The positive effects of time off from work, of being able to completely leave the cares and pressures (and even the positives) of the workplace behind, are by now too well-documented to ignore, as are the negative effects of burnout. The literature on vacations and recovery show that individuals, job performance, and companies all benefit from time out of the office. The most creative and most productive workers are the ones who are able to unplug from the office, recover their mental and physical energy, and return to their work recharged. We also now know that recovery isn't just a function of time off. We get the most from breaks when we do things that are relaxing, that let us experience control and mastery, and that provide a sense of detachment from our working lives. Recovery is active, not passive, and we can design it to get greater benefit.

The daily lives of creative workers have already shown us how they use early mornings and routines, walks, naps, and deliberate stops to stimulate their day-to-day creativity. When you take a wider view of their lives, you see a second pattern: that they use recovery experiences to sustain their creativity over long periods. Many of them are dedicated athletes: they find that exercise provides a break from work, strengthens the physical foundations of creative performance, and—as scientists have recently discovered—keeps their brains healthy. Deep play—hobbies that are challenging, mentally absorbing, and personally meaningful—provide another important source of recovery. Finally, sabbaticals give creative people a chance to reanimate their creative lives, explore new interests, and make life-changing breakthroughs. Together, they help intelligent, ambitious people stay curious, engaged, and productive, and help them lead long creative lives.

Exercise

> I hope that . . . the ideal of the well-trained and
> vigorous body will be maintained neck by neck with
> that of the well-trained and vigorous mind, as the
> two coequal halves of the higher education, for men
> and women alike.
>
> —WILLIAM JAMES

IN THE LATE 1950s, UCLA sociologist Bernice Eiduson
wanted to understand what separates great scientists from
their less-accomplished colleagues. Lots of psychologists had
tried to figure out what marked some people for greatness,
but no one had found the thing—the single personality trait,
the "genius gene," the cognitive edge—that all successful scientists share. Eiduson thought that by watching their careers
unfold over several decades and talking to and testing them
at regular intervals, she might see things in successful lives
that couldn't be identified through one-off interviews and

short studies. Eiduson found forty young and mid-career scientists at UCLA, Caltech, and elsewhere who agreed to be interviewed about their life and work, sit for psychological tests, and, most crucially, keep doing so. All of them were products of top graduate programs, promising researchers, and young enough to look forward to long, productive careers.

Eiduson followed this group for more than twenty years, and in that time the paths of the forty diverged. Some were elected to the prestigious National Academy of Sciences and received promotions and prestigious chairs at their universities. One became a presidential science advisor. Four won the Nobel Prize; one, Linus Pauling, won two. Others, in contrast, settled into less-distinguished careers. Some continued to struggle to do serious science but couldn't keep up. They became administrators or focused on teaching.

From a sociological standpoint, it was an ideal outcome. A group that looked roughly the same decades earlier had split into two parts. The challenge now was to figure out why.

The psychological profiles in Eiduson's group were maddeningly diverse. Their intelligence tests didn't routinely reveal inborn genius. There were some personality traits that good scientists shared—they had a high tolerance for uncertainty and lots of self-control, saw themselves as intellectual rebels, and maintained strong boundaries between home and work—but these traits aren't exactly rare. After Eiduson died in 1985, her longtime UCLA collaborator Maurine Bernstein kept the study going, joined by her son, Robert Scott Root-Bernstein, and statistician Helen Garnier. The three added some new questions to the interviews. They started asking the scientists whether they played sports or spent time outdoors. They asked about their hobbies and artistic interests. They asked how nonscientific activities connected or competed with each other. They asked how they managed their time and how pressed for time they felt.

The new questions revealed something interesting. The best scientists showed "an unusual urge to experiment athletically as well as scientifically" and selected "athletic activities that could be carried from youth into old age." Los Angeles conjures images of endless urban sprawl, but in fact the area is surrounded by hills and national parks, and thanks to its mild climate you can spend time outdoors most of the year. The top scientists took full advantage of the region's geography: they played tennis and went swimming, hiking, and skiing. This being Southern California, there was also an overrepresentation of surfers and sailors. Lots of them also walked regularly (no surprise). Their less-distinguished colleagues, in contrast, reported low rates of participation in sports. Some had played team sports in high school or college but gave them up after college and didn't take up something new.

One reason the findings of Bernstein, Root-Bernstein, and Garnier are striking is that they challenge the belief that intellectual activity and athletic ability are mutually exclusive. Terms like "vita contemplativa" or "life of the mind" don't exactly conjure up images of physical prowess, and they tap into a medieval belief that cultivation of the mind and spirit requires a denial of the body. Economists' classifications of "white-collar" versus "blue-collar" jobs, "knowledge work" versus manual labor, and knowledge-based economies versus ones that produce mere stuff, all tell us that work divides into neat, separate categories. In the United States, the notion that integrals and intervals don't mix is reinforced by American stereotypes about collegiate athletics and the unfortunate willingness of some sports-mad universities to tolerate underprepared student athletes while discouraging bright ones from pursuing academically demanding majors.

Despite this, a number of professional athletes have had distinguished academic careers. In the United States, professional football has had three Rhodes Scholars: Byron "Whizzer" White, who played for the Pittsburgh Pirates and the Detroit Lions in the 1930s (he later became a Supreme Court justice); Pat Haden, who played for the Los Angeles Rams in the 1970s; and Myron Rolle, who played for the Tennessee Titans and Pittsburgh Steelers from 2010 to 2012 before going to medical school. Frank Ryan, who played for the Cleveland Browns in the 1960s, received a PhD in math from Rice in 1965; more recently, mathematician and offensive lineman John Urschel published his first article on computational mathematics during his second season with the Baltimore Ravens and in 2016 started graduate work in applied mathematics at MIT. The NBA has had two Rhodes Scholars: Bill Bradley, who also won a gold medal as a member of the 1964 US Olympic basketball team and spent a decade with the New York Knicks before entering politics, and Tom McMillen, who played for the New York Knicks and Atlanta Hawks.

Conversely, a number of accomplished scientists have been noted athletes. The Danish physicist Niels Bohr and his mathematician brother, Harald, were both nationally ranked soccer players; Harald played for the Danish national team that won a silver medal at the 1908 Olympic games. Marie Curie, who shared the Nobel Prize in Physics in 1903 and won her own prize for Chemistry in 1911, was an avid cyclist: she and her husband, Pierre, went on a cycling tour on their honeymoon. America's first Olympic champion (for the 110-meter hurdle in 1896) was MIT electrical engineer Thomas Pelham Curtis, who went on to invent the modern electric toaster and blender. Roger Bannister was a medical student in 1954 when he became the first man to run a mile in under four minutes. He went on to a distinguished career as a neurologist. John Bardeen, who shared the 1956 Nobel Prize in Physics for his codiscovery of the transistor and the 1972 prize for his work on superconductivity, swam and played water polo in college and was an avid golfer. Cambridge biochemist Frederick Sanger, who won the 1958 Nobel Prize in Chemistry for developing a method for sequencing proteins, and shared the 1980 prize for his work on DNA sequencing, played rugby, football, and cricket in his youth, then switched to squash as an adult. Annette Salmeen won a gold medal in swimming for the United States at the 1996 Olympic games in Atlanta before studying neuroscience as a Rhodes Scholar at Oxford. Sarah Gerhardt became the first woman to surf the Mavericks, one of the world's most challenging and dangerous surf breaks in the world, while completing a PhD in physical chemistry.

The idea that academic and athletic excellence are mutually exclusive is also challenged by the existence of intellectual worlds that took sports very seriously and saw them as mutually supportive.

One of the greatest expressions of this philosophy can be found among the Cambridge "wranglers" during the nineteenth century. Academic accomplishment in nineteenth-century Cambridge was defined largely by performance on the Tripos, a weeklong series of exams required for third-year students. The Tripos was designed to be grueling: its nine exams grew increasingly devilish as the week unfolded, and you were graded both on how well you answered questions and how many questions you were able to answer. In other words, it rewarded accuracy, stamina, and an ability to work fast. A top performance opened the door to college fellowships and plum jobs, and bathed graduates in the glow of a bright future.

It was a system designed to test students; it could also break them. Some cracked in the examination hall and had to be carried out by their friends (who immediately rushed back to their desks). Even future scientific titans found preparing for the exams nerve-racking. William Thomson, the future Lord Kelvin (the temperature scale is named for him), and James Clerk Maxwell, who worked out the equations demonstrating that electricity and magnetism are two versions of the same phenomenon, both nearly broke under the pressure. Francis Galton, the future statistician and an influential popularizer of Darwin's (or as Galton called him, "cousin Charles") theory of evolution, had a nervous breakdown studying for the Tripos.

To avoid such a fate, ambitious students hired tutors to help them prepare for the Tripos, sometimes working with them for a solid two years. As the exams became tougher in the early nineteenth century, tutors began recommending students take long walks to get into shape before the exams. Walking was hardly unusual in Cambridge, but students aiming for top scores "transformed the traditional afternoon ramble or promenade into a daily regimen of measured physical exercise," according to historian Andrew Warwick. The most ambitious students became the most dedicated athletes, driven by a belief that "hard study was most efficiently and safely accomplished when interspersed with periods of more leisurely activity and recreation." Warwick found that for most of the nineteenth century, nearly "every high wrangler . . . participated in some form of regular physical exercise to preserve his physical strength and stamina." Rowing was especially popular because it taught you how to deliver a consistent, "machine-like regularity of performance" on the river, and in the examination hall. Not only did they see exercise as the "complement of hard study," students even tried out "different regimes of working, exercising and sleeping until they found what they believed to be the most productive combination." You don't self-experiment like this if you want to fit in. You're trying to stand out. To be outstanding.

The connection between academic study and athletic training lives on in another Cambridge legacy. The tutors came to be famous for driving their students along well-set paths, working on progressively harder problems, with the aim of emerging victorious in competition. A well-run tutorial, students said, was like a team of horses led by a coachman—or, as Cambridge students came to call their tutors, a "coach."

Another, more informal example of an athletically vigorous world-class scientific community is the laboratory of Oxford neuroscientist Charles Sherrington. Sherrington was one of the founders of modern neuroscience: he coined the term *synapse*, won a share of the 1932 Nobel Prize in Physiology or Medicine, and his students, who came from all over the world, helped create our modern understanding of the brain. They identified and named its major structures, mapped its regions, developed instruments to follow signals as they moved between brain and muscles, and turned brain surgery from a ghoulish last resort into a surgical specialty. Three would win Nobel Prizes.

Charles Sherrington studied medicine at St. Thomas's Hospital in London and graduated from Cambridge in 1885. Small but powerful, he was a ferocious rugby player and rower; this early athleticism gave him "a strong constitution which enabled him to carry out prolonged researches," as his Nobel biography put it. As a professor at Liverpool and Oxford, Sherrington displayed a preference for students who were both scientists and sportsmen. This made his laboratory a favorite destination for Rhodes Scholars. One of his first, Wilder Penfield, was class president and football tackle at Princeton; after graduating he deferred his Rhodes Scholarship for a year (until 1914) to coach the Princeton football team. Australian Howard Florey had played tennis, cricket, and football in school. Despite a comfortable childhood, at Oxford he "endeavored to look like the hardened criminal of the bush everyone expected," Florey told a friend back home. But he quickly proved to be an outstanding student, and at Sherrington's urging he went on to take a D.Phil at Cambridge. John Farquhar Fulton arrived in early 1923 from Harvard; he quickly proved to be a savvy academic player and prolific writer, speeding through the D.Phil in two years and dazzling Sherrington as "an artist in research." Sherrington's last Rhodes Scholar, Australian John Eccles, arrived at Oxford in 1923 with a medical degree from the University of Melbourne and an armful of track-and-field prizes.

Another of Sherrington's students, Thomas Graham Brown, achieved renown not as a neurophysiologist—Sherrington actually thought him a bit of a disappointment—but as the first person to climb the Brenva face of Mont Blanc. Brown became part of a third community of scientist-athletes: mountain climbers. The mountains have attracted many of the century's great scientists: Marie Curie and Albert Einstein went hiking together in the Alps. Neils Bohr, Hans Bethe, Enrico Fermi, and Edward Teller hiked in the Alps as students and in the mountains around Los Alamos while working on the Manhattan Project. For some, the beauty of a summit and the opportunity to commune with nature gave mountain climbing a legitimacy other sports lacked. In high school in Vienna during the 1920s, MIT physicist Victor Weisskopf recalled, the self-styled intellectuals were avid hikers and skiers who rationalized that "they were not really sports" because mountain sports "involved something much higher, the love of nature." Rosalind Franklin, the X-ray crystallographer whose work helped James Watson and Francis

Crick discover the double-helical structure of DNA, discovered mountain climbing as a teen, when her family went glacier climbing in Norway. Later, as a postdoc in Paris, where she mastered X-ray crystallography, she moved from hiking to more-technical climbs during frequent trips to the French and Italian Alps. By the time she returned to England and King's College, London, she was as confident on peaks as in the lab. The mountains of Southern California attracted émigré astronomers Rudolph Minkowski and Fritz Zwicky (who coined the term *supernova*) to Caltech. Climbing continues to be a favorite pastime of physicists: UC Santa Barbara physicist Steve Giddings, an expert on black holes and quantum gravity, is an avid mountain and ice climber, while Harvard string theorist Lisa Randall's climbing exploits have been commemorated with a Lisa Randall Wall in Colorado, a sixty-foot granite climb in the mountains outside Denver.

IRONICALLY, FOR ALL their interest in sports, none of Sherrington's students ever investigated the effect of exercise on cognitive performance and the brain. However, this has been an active field in recent decades. At first, researchers mainly investigated the benefits of exercise for healthy aging, but studies now show that for people of any age, gender, or athletic ability, exercise can increase brain power, boost intelligence, and provide the stamina and psychological resilience necessary to do creative work.

Studies of the effects of fitness programs on brain structure and health have shown that exercise improves brain structure, just as it does the cardiovascular system and muscles.

In a 2015 German and Finnish study, before-and-after brain scans of overweight and obese subjects showed dramatic improvement in the volume of grey matter and white matter over the course of a three-month fitness and weight loss program. Exercise doesn't just make your brain healthier by reducing cholesterol or improving cardiovascular capacity; exercise actually "induces profound structural brain plasticity."

Scientists have begun to work out the specific mechanisms connecting exercise and brain development. In particular, they've focused on the role that exercise plays in boosting the production of neurotrophins, proteins that encourage the formation and growth of neurons. For years scientists have known that brain-derived neurotrophic factor, or BDNF, triggers the development of new neurons. But what triggers the generation of BDNF? In 2013, Harvard Medical School researchers found that in mice, the hormone irisin stimulates the brain to produce BDNF; irisin, in turn, is generated by the muscles during endurance exercise. Not long after that, a team at Boston University found elevated levels of BDNF in the blood of physically fit students.

Running seems to be particularly effective in stimulating neurogenesis. Scientists have found that mice running on wheels generate twice the number of new neurons in their hippocampus as mice who are sedentary; they are also better able to identify new objects and distinguish similar objects from one another. A comparative study showed that rats who ran on a running wheel showed higher levels of neurogenesis than rats who went through a program of resistance training (climbing a wall while carrying a weight) and high-intensity interval training (alternately sprinting and walking on a treadmill).

Exercise generally has indirect but positive effects on creativity. Since the 1960s, studies have found that a session of aerobic exercise can have a small but direct effect on creativity among people who are in good shape. In one 2005 study, for example, physically fit college-age students were given the Torrance creativity test immediately after and then two hours after thirty minutes of aerobic exercise; all tested higher than when they hadn't exercised. But people who don't normally exercise don't get the same creative boost from a workout. In 2013, a team of researchers found that athletes' scores on a convergent-thinking test went up slightly after exercising, but exercise impaired the performance of nonathletes. If you're a couch potato, a spin class or a 10K right before a brainstorming session will be exhausting, not energizing.

These findings are in keeping with writers' and scientists' own reports of the role of strenuous exercise in their creative lives. Murakami took up long-distance running after finishing his second novel, and "it was my belated, but real, starting point as a novelist," he says, but he doesn't think about plotlines while on the road. "What exactly do I think about when I'm running? I don't have a clue," he says. "I run in a void." A long walk or hike can stimulate new ideas in the moment; a long run stimulates ideas afterward and improves your ability to turn good ideas into creative works.

Aerobic activity is beneficial in several ways. Exercise strengthens your cardiovascular system and improves your circulation, which means your body can deliver more blood to your brain when it's working. Because the brain's demand for oxygen and sugar rises when you're concentrating hard, this can make the difference between grasping that insight or feeling like it's just out of reach. A firing neuron uses as much energy as a leg muscle cell during a marathon. Further, sustained aerobic exercise stimulates the body to generate more small blood vessels in the brain, and a better-developed cerebral vasculature can deliver blood to the brain faster and more effectively. A 2012 study found that episodic memory improves as maximal oxygen capacity increases. (Conversely, comparative studies of adults who do and don't exercise find that couch potatoes have lower scores on tests of executive function and processing speed and in middle age have faster rates of brain aging and memory decline.)

Physical stamina is also as important for creative work as for manual labor. We often underestimate how physically demanding cognitive tasks can be, especially ones that require focus for hours at a time, but as novelist Haruki Murakami puts it, "finishing an entire book is closer to manual labor" and "requires far more energy, over a long period, than most people ever imagine." He trains for marathons because it helps build the concentration and stamina to write. Japanese stem cell researcher Shinya Yamanaka, who compares the challenges of world-class science to marathon running, ran a 4:03 in the Tokyo Marathon in 2012, the same year he won a share of the Nobel Prize in Physiology or Medicine for his work on induced pluripotent stem (iPS) cells. MIT professor Wolfgang Ketterle, who won a share of the 2011 Nobel Prize in Physics for his work on Bose–Einstein condensates, posted a 2:44 at the 2014 Boston Marathon. World-class chess players now work as intensively in the gym as they do on the chessboard. Chess has always been mentally demanding, but in an era of computer-enhanced training and high-stakes international tournaments, players must be able to focus intensely for longer periods than ever. Physical and mental stamina is now essential for world-class play. In 1995, when preparing for a twenty-game match, Viswanathan Anand went on long walks after studying games; twenty years later, his training regimen included cycling, a one-kilometer swim, and a ten-kilometer run. Magnus Carlsen, one of the highest-rated masters in the history of the game, famously spends hours a day on the treadmill and weight machines.

Regular exercise also relieves stress and increases your capacity to deal with the pressures of difficult jobs. A study of the off-hours of self-professed workaholics found that those who engage in physically strenuous activity are happier than those who engage in more passive leisure. In his study of burnout among American surgeons, Tait Shanafelt found that regular exercise is a significant predictor of higher quality of life. Workaholics are more likely than other people to feel anxiety about work when they're out of the office, and exercise provides an outlet for nervous energy and a different focus for mental energy. For people in high-stress jobs, it can be one of the few factors contributing to recovery that can be easily modified: it's much harder to change your marital status, family commitments, or income than to sign up for a spin class.

Strenuous exercise can retrain your body's reaction to stressors. Exposing yourself to predictable, incremental physical stressors in the gym or the playing field increases your capacity to be calm and clear-headed in stressful real-world situations. President Barack Obama maintained a strict fitness routine throughout his political career; according to his personal assistant, Reggie Love, daily workouts "were key to surviving" long campaigns and the rigors of governing. Elena Kagan took up boxing after joining the Supreme Court and is only the latest justice to develop an exercise regimen to deal with the demands of the high court. (In fact, she and Ruth Bader Ginsberg use the same personal trainer.) Mathematician and computer pioneer Alan Turing ran to get a break from his work: developing the first generation of electronic computers was, he said, "such a stressful job that the only way I can get it out of my mind is by running hard." UCLA chemist and Nobel laureate Donald Cram was an avid surfer: "being slammed down by a 10-ton avalanche of violent water" provided a "big release" of emotional and physical energy, he said, "allowing me to sit still for long periods of time."

When he was on Robben Island between 1962 and 1988, Nelson Mandela used exercise to combat the stresses of imprisonment. Prisoners at Robben Island were forced to do hard labor, making gravel and later working in a quarry, but maintaining a boxer's workout regimen (running in place for forty-five minutes, a hundred push-ups, and two hundred sit-ups) gave Mandela a way to take charge of his own captivity, to resist the government's efforts to control and break him, and to show that he would remain his own man. More practically, he later wrote, "I have always believed exercise is a key not only to physical health but to peace of mind" and "I worked better and thought more clearly when I was in good physical condition"—a kind of self-cultivation that benefited him and needled his captors. Consequently, "training became one of the inflexible disciplines of my life," and he continued with his morning workouts even after his release from prison.

Playing sports in your youth and staying athletic in adulthood can also have long-term benefits for your career and health. A study of Swedish military veterans found a positive correlation among cardiovascular fitness and intelligence test scores at eighteen, higher academic achievement a decade later, and higher incomes thirty years later. A 2014 study of the lives of American men who had been in high school before World War II found that veterans who had been athletes in high school went on to make more money, have higher-status careers, and become professionals and managers in greater numbers than those who did not. (They also spent more time doing volunteer work and gave more to charity.) Some of the advantage was self-fulfilling, the product of positive stereotypes: employers who assume that ex-athletes are natural leaders and have more self-confidence, self-respect, and grit tend to give ex-athletes more opportunities to develop and exhibit those capabilities, which sets them up for more success and more opportunities.

The impact of sports on the careers of businesswomen may be even stronger. In 2014, four hundred female executives were surveyed about their athletic experiences. Ninety-seven percent of the executives who had reached C-suite positions (that is, they had "chief" in their titles) had played sports at some point in their lives, 52 percent had played sports in college, and 53 percent still played some sport. Two-thirds said that they looked more favorably on prospective employees if they were athletes (there's the positive stereotype again), and almost as many said their athletic experience had been a factor in their success.

A number of large-scale studies have shown that physical activity can also slow cognitive decline. In 2015, scientists at King's College London published the results of a ten-year study of the relationship between physical activity and cognitive aging in twin sisters. Scientists argue over how much genetic, behavioral, and environmental factors affect things like aging, intelligence, and success; in studies comparing identical twins, genetics ceases to be a factor. The researchers administered psychological, neurological, and health and fitness tests to 324 twins in 1999 and again in 2009, with the aim of understanding how different factors affect changes in cognitive ability (determined using a battery of tests to measure memory and processing speed) and global brain structure. They also took MRI scans of subjects' brains. The study found that twins who were stronger and more physically active in 1999 did better on cognitive tests in 2009 and had better global brain structure, and that activity and strength had a "protective effect," slowing age-related cognitive change.

Another recent study revisited an old test to measure the effects of physical activity on the cognitive health of elderly

Scottish people. In the summer of 1947, social scientists administered intelligence tests to virtually every eleven-year-old in Scotland. Nearly sixty years later, scientists in Edinburgh tracked down a thousand members of this group, dusted off the old 1947 intelligence test (Moray House Test No. 12), and gave them a battery of new tests assessing their mental health, physical fitness, and so on; a couple years later, they all had MRIs. Now called the Lothian Birth Cohort 1936, the group is providing a wealth of information about the factors that affect the aging brain because their current test results can be compared to those of their eleven-year-old selves. In one article, scientists reported a positive correlation between levels of physical activity, connectivity between brain regions, and white matter quantity and density.

Other researchers have tracked the health and behavior of tens of thousands of nurses, British civil servants, and other groups over the course of years or decades, and have consistently observed a positive relationship between physical activity and healthy aging. Many of these studies have demonstrated that staying physically active in your forties and fifties—the period when you're likely to be busiest with family and work and when excuses to skip exercise come most easily—pays off for decades: exercising in midlife reduces the risk of chronic disease and dementia late in life. But you don't have to be an athlete in your forties to reap the cognitive and health benefits of exercise in your later years, as the example of Olga Kotelko shows. Kotelko was a Canadian athlete who won hundreds of senior track and field events before her death at ninety-four. Scientists found that her regimen had a dramatic effect on her brain's structure: compared to other people her age, Kotelko's brain had greater white matter integrity (which correlates with increased capacity for reasoning, self-control, and planning) and levels of fractional anisotropy (a measure of brain connectivity), and her healthier brain helped her perform better on cognition and memory tests. What makes this more remarkable is that while she had grown up on a farm and spent a career as a teacher, she didn't start competing until late in life: she started training at seventy-seven.

These studies help explain how some scientists, writers, painters, and architects manage to stay productive decades after the competition has burned out. The architect Le Corbusier was working on four projects when he died at seventy-seven during his regular afternoon swim; Charles Darwin spent his last afternoon on the Sandwalk a few weeks before his death at seventy-two. Sherrington and his students had remarkably long, distinguished careers. Wilder Penfield founded the Montreal Institute of Neurology, pioneered surgical techniques for treating epilepsy, and used electrical stimulation of the brain to develop the first functional map of the cerebral cortex. Howard Florey returned to Oxford in 1935 to run the Dunn School of Pathology, where he and Ernst Chain would lead the development of penicillin as an antibiotic. John Eccles stayed at Oxford until 1937, then returned to Australia, where his research on chemical and electrical signaling in the central nervous system won him a share of the 1963 Nobel Prize in Physiology or Medicine. All three spent long hours in the lab: Penfield sometimes had to spend days monitoring patients after surgery, Eccles's experiments often ran for thirty-six hours straight, and Florey's early work on penicillin required keeping the Dunn School working around the clock. But even through their busiest years, they remained avid athletes: they made time for tennis or sailing during weekends and vacations, or had extensive gardens (Florey even has a rose variety named after him). Given the value of midlife exercise in shaping health and cognitive activity in late life, it's no surprise that several continued publishing well into their eighties. Clearly the popular assumption that youthful genius can't last is true only if you want it to be.

John Fulton, who seemed the most promising of the group, serves as the cautionary tale. Unlike the others, he didn't handle the pressures of work by carving out time for rest or exercise; instead, he fell into drinking. By forty he was a high-functioning alcoholic, and eventually he lost his laboratory and professorship. He occasionally displayed some of his old brilliance as a writer, but after years of trying and failing to sober up, Fulton died at the age of sixty-one in 1960.

THE FINDINGS OF Bernice Eiduson and her collaborators and the examples of the Cambridge wranglers, Sherrington and his circle, scientist-climbers, and other scholar-athletes, offer some valuable lessons for people who need to balance busy schedules and creative lives. While Victorian gentleman naturalists, novelists, composers, and surrealist painters are models of creative success, their daily lives can sometimes seem a little too unconstrained to serve as useful models for today. Plenty of these figures were also good athletes (you can't walk ten miles a day, as Charles Dickens did regularly, without it benefitting you), but many of the lives of athletically inclined scientists, doctors, and politicians bear a more obvious resemblance to our own. Successful scientists are super busy people. At the best of times, you only have to write grant proposals, teach undergraduates, mentor graduate students, manage your lab, and help run your department— and, when you have the time, do science. If you work in a corporate R & D lab or start-up, the stack of obligations is different but just as tall. And the more prominent you are, the more committees, panels, conferences, working groups, and reviews you're asked to take on.

A successful career in science, in other words, attracts distractions like a magnet attracts iron filings. The daily lives of the scientists in Eiduson's study look more like those of surgeons or lawyers than of novelists. Their calendars were hemmed in by deadlines, weighed down by committees, and carved up by bosses (not to mention kids, family, and everything else). But the best of them were able to make the time to get out of the lab on a regular basis to go hiking or surfing or rock climbing, to play tennis or run. They defied the stereotypes of nerdy, weak scientists, and they reaped the benefits. Even though it doesn't directly use muscle power, intellectual and professional labor is physically challenging: staying focused for hours at a time, switching attention from research to administration, moving from surgical theater to meeting room, takes stamina. Likewise, it's valuable for helping deal with the pressures and disappointments of professional life. It helps you live a longer, healthier life. And it helps you maintain your intellectual edge and creative powers for more of your life.

When we think of work and rest as opposites, or treat exercise as something that would be good to do when we finally have the time, we risk becoming like the low achievers in Eiduson's group. Exercise helped Eiduson's stars, and many other high-achieving communities, have long productive lives. We shouldn't be surprised that people manage to be physically active and do world-class work. We should recognize that they do world-class work because they are physically active.

Deep Play

The cultivation of a hobby and new forms of interest is therefore a policy of first importance to a public man.

—Winston Churchill

THE MAKER FAIRE is one of the more remarkable fixtures of Silicon Valley life. An annual gathering of engineers, tinkerers, high-tech artists, craftspeople, and science and technology educators, the scene is a cross between a county fair, an MIT faculty meeting, and a jubilant space shuttle launch. Homemade steampunk clothing and developer-conference fleece pullovers are the uniforms of choice. You can enjoy fried food and cotton candy, test out some home-brew shotgun genomics, and watch 3-D printers make everything from chocolate to circuits. The exhibits are a wonderful mix of high-tech found art and Arduino microcontrollers. One subset of exhibitors seems determined to put flamethrowers on anything that moves, and most things that don't. In a weekend, the Faire uses enough propane to warm the hearts of OPEC accountants. If the Mad Max universe had Etsy, it would look like this.

Towering over the scene is an eighteen-foot-tall, one-ton robot giraffe named Russell. The Electric Giraffe is the Maker Faire's biggest celebrity, both figuratively and literally. Children flock to him, alternately mesmerized and energized. He responds when they pet him: stroke the touch-activated sensors on his nose, and his lights flash and he chirps and beeps. The effect doesn't get old, partly because he's different every Faire: his builder, Lindsay Lawlor, tinkers with the 'Raffe throughout the year, improving the controls and making him more responsive. Seeing him at the Faire is like catching up with an old acquaintance: part of the pleasure of the encounter is seeing how you've both changed.

Like all animals, the Giraffe evolved to thrive in a specific environment: Burning Man, the annual art festival / utopian city / retreat / rave that takes place on the Playa, a huge dry lake bed, in Black Rock, Nevada. One year Lawlor, who had attended Burning Man dressed in a zebra costume, realized that a walking robot giraffe would fit right in with the art bikes and art cars (register with the Department of Mutant Vehicles) that roam the open space. If you really want to build something that grabs attention, it helps to be well-lit: many of the artworks and experimental architecture are most dazzling at night. On a flat, featureless plain, being tall gets attention. It also means that the view from even a slight elevation—like riding atop a giraffe—is stunning.

In late 2004 Lawlor started building. He would come home from work, head into the machine shop in his garage, and spend the evening working on the giraffe; on the weekends he would be in the shop eight or ten hours a day, welding parts, testing motors, fixing gears. In the last month before Burning Man 2005, he was "up until three or four in the morning working on it."

The Electric Giraffe started out as a side project, but a one-ton robot has a way of taking on a life of its own. In the years since, Lawlor has continued improving it. "It's not like restoring a '57 Chevy," which has an ideal, original state, he says; it's more like "an endless canvas that you can keep changing and working on." On one visit to Maker Faire, you might see new lights and sensors on his head and neck; another year, the motion sensors have been upgraded. Every year the Giraffe is a little different, a little more interactive, and a little more interesting.

The Electric Giraffe illustrates how some hobbies are much more than a diversion. Under the right conditions, hobbies and physical activities become what anthropologists and psychologists call "deep play," activities that are rewarding on their own, but take on additional layers of meaning and personal significance. Play is one of the most important things we do. Children and young animals refine essential skills through play: children learn how to cooperate, follow rules, expand their imaginations, strengthen body and mind, and take failure in stride. Because play is voluntary, intrinsically rewarding, mentally and physically engaging, and imaginative, it's often absorbing and effortless; even when it's physically challenging or uncomfortable, it's not difficult in the same way a hard day at work is.

The term *deep play* was popularized by anthropologist Clifford Geertz, in a now-classic article about the deep meaning of Balinese cockfighting. Simple games of chance, like dice or three-card monte, and very simple video games aren't deep; they provide a momentary pleasure or distraction, but shallow games don't teach you skills that you can use in life, nor do they reveal much about your character. Deep play, in contrast, is about much more than the game. In Bali, cockfighting allows displays of wealth and social status, ritualized competition between villages, and acts of personal violence and rage that would be taboo elsewhere. When it's competitive, deep play has high symbolic stakes. When it's personal, it offers lasting benefits and satisfaction that shallow play does not.

In creative lives, activities become deep play when they have at least one of four features.

First, deep play is mentally absorbing. It offers the player challenges to face and problems to solve. Like all recovery experiences, that engagement doesn't require effort; the player falls into the game easily. It may give the player the chance to learn new things, or discover things about themselves, that they would not in their work.

Second, deep play offers players a new context in which to use some of the same skills that they use in their work. If using those skills well is a pleasure, it's not surprising that people would enjoy using them both in their work and in their leisure. Indeed, finding them useful in a new game can provide its own gratification.

Third, deep play offers some of the same satisfaction as work, but it also offers different, clearer rewards thanks to differences in media or scale or pace. Ben Kazez's description of app development and musical performance as requiring collaboration with smart people, interacting with audiences, and making choices in interpretation and performance is one example of finding similar rewards in different domains. Researchers used to open-ended problems and leaders managing in uncertain times may find deep play in activities with finite horizons, clear boundaries, and unambiguous rules and rewards. For scientists and writers who labor for years on projects, games that can be accomplished in a few days can be deeply satisfying. Scientists used to thinking at the subatomic or cosmic scale may take pleasure in confronting a human-sized challenge.

Finally, deep play provides a living connection to the player's past. It may build on things the player did with parents, have features that remind the player of a childhood home or activities from the player's youth, or in other ways serve as a way of keeping links with the past alive.

This combination of absorption, use of skills in new contexts, similar satisfactions through different means, and personal connection makes deep play a powerful break from work, a respite from professional frustrations, and a source of recovery. Deep play becomes worthwhile because its rewards are so substantial. Deep play can acquire momentum, pulling its players in directions they never expected to go.

Creative people don't engage in deep play despite their high levels of activity and productivity; they're active and productive because of deep play.

FOR A YEAR, Norman Maclean, then a first-year graduate student at the University of Chicago, played billiards with the elderly Albert Michelson in the university's Quadrangle Club in 1928. At the time, Michelson was one of the best-known scientists in America. The first American to win a Nobel Prize (in Physics in 1907), Michelson had designed a series of instruments that measured the speed of light with unprecedented accuracy. His first great experiments, conducted with his colleague Edward Morley in the 1880s, later became famous as history's most important failed experiment. Physicists had assumed that light waves, radio waves, and other electromagnetic radiation traveled through the "luminiferous ether," much as waves travel through water. Michelson and Morley had calculated that by making an interferometer that split a beam of light into two parts and sent them off at ninety-degree angles to each other, they would be able to detect changes in the speed of light as the two beams moved with or against the ether's motion. Instead, they could detect no change at all. But the experiment was so well-designed and clear that it was seen as a blow against the theory of the ether and helped clear the way for Einstein's theory of general relativity.

The Michelson-Morley experiment became a landmark in the history of science, but it nearly destroyed Michelson. In the middle of his research, Michelson had a nervous breakdown: months of overwork on nerve-rackingly delicate instruments, financial and personal problems, and his employer's indifference to his research combined to leave him exhausted. Three months in a sanitarium allowed him to return to work, but now he was more mindful of his energy and made a deliberate effort to rest. He took up tennis, becoming one of the first Americans to master a topspin stroke, and walked in the afternoons after teaching and laboratory work. He also sought recovery in activities from his youth. Michelson had grown up in a mining town in the Sierra Nevada mountains of California in the 1850s. During the Gold Rush such towns attracted "many cultivated men seeking a fortune, among them a fine violinist who taught little Albert," as his wife recalled. Now, he resumed playing the violin every morning, and he would continue to do so for the rest of his life. In the summers he took up painting and sailing, both of which he had studied at the US Naval Academy.

Later, when age caught up with him on the tennis court, he switched to billiards. Why billiards? When he first saw Michelson play, Maclean recognized the kind of figure he had grown up watching in the local saloon in Montana in the early 1900s. Michelson even looked the part: "slight, trim and handsome," dressed in "a high, stiff collar and a small, sharp mustache," he would have fit right in at the Card and Billiards Emporium.

Michelson turned to deep play to maintain the energy and psychological reserves necessary to build almost unimaginably precise instruments that could measure changes in fractions of a wavelength of light. His choices reflected both his upbringing and talent. It's easy to imagine the violin or pool cue stirring occasional memories of the mining town of his childhood, with its European fortune-seekers and saloons. But Michelson was also the "best head-and-hands man in the world," as Maclean put it, and it was natural that he would take pleasure in games "involving something like a cue, a brush, a bow, or, best of all, a box with slits and silvered mirrors," and see all those games as building on and improving each other.

Painting was also deep play for Winston Churchill. Churchill took up painting in 1915, after resigning from the Admiralty over the Gallipoli disaster and finding himself (not for the last time in his life) on the outside of events he desperately wanted to influence. He explained the appeal of the art in a small book helpfully titled *Painting as a Pastime*. Busy people need to cultivate forms of rest, he began, but are temperamentally unable to simply do nothing. "It is not enough merely to switch off the lights which play upon the main and ordinary field of interest," he argued. "A new field of interest must be illuminated." Fortunately, "the tired parts of the mind can be rested and strengthened, not merely by rest, but by using other parts."

Churchill found painting a valuable pastime for several reasons. It required complete concentration, but it was an easy-to-achieve focus. "I know of nothing which, without exhausting the body, more entirely absorbs the mind," he said. "Whatever the worries of the hour or the threats of the future, once the picture has begun to flow along, there is no room for them." It offered an inexhaustible supply of new subjects, new skills to master, and a lifetime of challenges. "Every step may be fruitful. Yet there will stretch out before you an ever-lengthening, ever-ascending, ever-improving path."

Painting also had some of the qualities that made military and political life so appealing. "In all battles two things are usually required of the Commander-in-Chief: to make a good plan for his army and, secondly, to keep a strong reserve. Both these are also obligatory upon the painter." Painting "is like fighting a battle," he wrote, or "unfolding a long, sustained, interlocked argument. It is a proposition which, whether of few or numberless parts, is commanded by a single unity of conception." A large canvas by J. M. W. Turner is the "equal in quality and intensity of the finest achievements of warlike action." Both battles and paintings required careful study of the problem before them, informed by "the achievements of the great Captains of the past" on the battlefield or in the gallery.

At the same time, he found, painting was also different from politics. "Just to paint is great fun. The colors are lovely to look at and delicious to squeeze out." This physicality made it a pleasant change from a daily grind of reading reports, responding to memos, and attending meetings.

Churchill's description of the appeal of painting is highly personal. Few painters would see themselves as similar to commanders or orators. But it makes an important point: that connections between work and deep play are made by individuals and don't just exist, waiting to be found.

Sailing is another popular form of deep play. For scientists and engineers, it calls on the same problem-solving and observational skills they use at work, but in briefer, more intense, and more physical bursts. For industrial designer Jack Kelley, who invented the first mouse pad and helped create the modern cubicle, weekend races on Lake Michigan "refreshed [his] thought process" as design director at office furniture company Herman Miller. The Victorian physicist William Thomson, whose work on thermodynamics and electromagnetism helped rewrite nineteenth-century physics, spent most of his summers on his yacht, the *Lalla Rookh*. He was an excellent sailor but also described the yacht as "the quietest and best place attainable for work," and he would retreat to it when working on difficult problems.

Sailing was an even deeper form of play for biophysicist Britton Chance, who wrote or coauthored fifteen hundred articles, was awarded over two hundred patents, and won a gold medal in sailing at the 1952 Olympics in Helsinki. For Chance, sailing was a family activity: he learned to sail with his father and taught each of his own eleven children. It was also another venue for exercising his technical ingenuity: as a teen he invented an automatic ship-steering mechanism, and as an adult he developed a system (promptly outlawed by race officials) that injected drag-reducing long-chain polymers in the water ahead of his yacht. Finally, it was mentally restorative. Weekend races provided a much-needed break from his sixty-hour weeks as head of the Johnson Foundation at the University of Pennsylvania: one student recalled that conversation "switched from nearly all science to nearly all sailing" on the drive from Philadelphia to New Jersey's Barnegat Bay. Training for the 1952 Olympics provided an even longer and equally fruitful respite. After years of focusing on work, he later said, it was a period when "sailing took complete priority over science." But instead of slowing his career, the break "helped invigorate my research. Having conquered the waters, I was ready for an even bigger challenge, tackling the great unknowns of biochemistry."

Scientists who become renowned both in the laboratory and on mountain peaks practice an especially rigorous form of deep play. In contrast to their holiday-making peers, for whom climbing is a form of vigorous nature-worship, these climbers treat the sport as a platform for innovation and record-setting activity. Exploring new climbing techniques and climbing in more-remote and difficult terrain means spending significant time and energy on what colleagues might regard as a distraction. So what makes the investment worth it? The answer is that undertaking harder, more daring climbs allows for more complete absorption and allows them to discover stronger connections between their climbing and science.

Unlike a long walk or hike, which can be an occasion for mind-wandering, mountain climbing requires absolute focus. Viktor Frankl, the Austrian psychotherapist and author of the classic *Man's Search for Meaning*, said, "My hours spent in climbing were the only ones during which I gave no thought to my next lecture or book." In a life defined by patients, lectures, and books, "when I reached the wall . . . you [would] not find me thinking of anything but the climbing. . . . I was prohibited from thinking about my next book or anything else." Christof Koch, director of the Allen Institute for Brain Science in Seattle and one of the world's leading neuroscientists, describes a similar experience: "You're out there on the edge, you're out there on the sharp end of a rope, and you're hyper-conscious of the world," he says. "It's a form of meditation because you are engaged to such an extent with the world, with the environment, you have to

208

pay such attention to every little unevenness in the rock, that your inner voice—this constant critic that's always in your head—is completely silent."

Elite mountain climbing requires some of the same problem-solving skills that scientists use in their work. Physicist Henry Kendall, who won a share of the 1990 Nobel Prize for his experiments demonstrating the existence of quarks, brought some of his experimental genius from the laboratory when, along with other Stanford climbers in the 1950s, he helped create a new style of free climbing that emphasized natural handholds and used ropes for safety rather than support; decades later he invented one of the pitons used in ice climbing. Kendall was also one of the first to carry a portable camera on his climbs and to take pictures during a climb; the pictures he took of Yosemite in the late 1950s make Kendall the sport's equivalent of Robert Capa or Ansel Adams. Kendall drew a parallel between photography and mountain climbing on one hand and physics on the other in a Nobel address. He enjoyed exploring "places no one has been before," whether mountain peaks or atomic nuclei. "The world is an astonishingly beautiful place. It is beautiful at the deep level of physics, way down inside things," he said, and "the universe that is visible to us is also of astonishing beauty, and I like to see that and explore it. That is why I take photographs." John Gill, a professor of mathematics at the University of Southern Colorado, pioneered the modern sport of rock climbing—the variety practiced now on indoor climbing walls—by borrowing from gymnastics to create a more dynamic, fluid style of climbing, and advancing the idea that a technically challenging, world-class climb could happen ten feet off the ground. He sees deep similarities between climbing and mathematics. In both fields, you're always searching for "an interesting result—ideally an unexpected result—in an elegant fashion, with a smooth flow, using some unexpected simplicity." When you begin a climb, "you stand upon the threshold of something new, something that requires not only brute force (whether it be physical or intellectual force) but a certain insight, a certain quantum jump from point to point." Finally, the "reward, in both activities, is almost continual enlightenment."

For Louis Reichardt, "climbing a route is in some ways like designing an experiment;" in both cases, "you don't even know what you have to know to solve the problem in many cases. And so you just take it a step at a time, and use your best judgment and hope for the best." Reichardt started climbing as a graduate student at Stanford in the 1960s and developed a reputation as one of the world's experts on the brain (he studies neurotrophins and other proteins that keep the brain running) and as "one of the most powerful, capable, and determined mountaineers in the world" virtually simultaneously. Reichardt was notable for establishing new paths up hard-to-reach mountains. In 1973, he climbed Nepal's Dhaulagiri, the seventh-tallest mountain in the world, spending more than three weeks above 7,800 meters and reaching the summit without supplemental oxygen. In 1981 he was part of the first American team to climb K2; two years later he summited Mount Everest from the eastern face (a route that even Edmund Hillary had refused to try, declaring that "others more foolish might try this, but it was not for us"). Given the months required to plan expeditions in the Himalayas, it was impossible to imagine repeating a route; "just like in science, you try to do something new. You try to do something that is not in other people's footsteps." But without the challenge, without the prospect of failure, neither would be as rewarding.

On the other hand, strenuous climbing is also different. For Henry Kendall, part of the appeal of mountains is that "they can be appreciated on a large scale in quite striking contrast to the microscopic things I study professionally." In contrast to physics, success in climbing is quick and decisive. It can take years for ambitious, complicated physics experiments to get funded and finished, and even then the results may be ambiguous. Climbs are shorter and their results unambiguous: either you solve the various problems before you and make it to the summit or you don't. Even if the route is obscure or difficult, the goal is very clear.

Finally, climbing provides a perspective that can be elusive in the competitive world of science. Herbert de Staebler, a friend of Kendall's and fellow climber, said that climbers like Kendall had "skill, the physical stamina and strength," but also mental toughness: "Confidence is such a feeble word to describe what it takes to operate at those levels." Nick Clinch, another of Kendall's contemporaries, noted that on the mountains, you were "hit with more sense of responsibility . . . than you have in almost any other student thing you can be doing." Having "people's lives at stake" provided a "sense of responsibility and maturity" that most students never developed. As Reichardt put it, it teaches the difference between disappointing experiences, like having a grant turned down, and "the truly devastating," like losing a fellow climber. Setbacks in the laboratory, he said, "simply didn't have the same consequences . . . as what had happened in the mountains."

THERE ARE ALSO some forms of deep play that go on for decades and ultimately turn into second careers or produce unexpected masterpieces.

Neurosurgeon Wilder Penfield began a second career as a writer after he retired from the Montreal Institute of Neurology in 1960 at age seventy. Between then and his death in 1976, he wrote two novels and four works of nonfiction. Yet his life as a writer had been incubating for decades. From his freshman year at Princeton in 1909 to his mother's death in 1943, he had written her faithfully, and through this correspondence—over a thousand letters in which he described his studies, travels, and family life—he acquired the habits of a regular writer. His first novel was actually one that she had started and he rewrote and completed. In a sense, Penfield never stopped writing to his mother. Even his most technical book, *Mystery of the Mind*, was subtly autobiographical: it dealt with questions about the relationship between mind and brain that he had first encountered more than sixty years earlier as a student at Princeton and had pondered ever since. It was dedicated to his mentor, Charles Sherrington.

In an era of text messaging and e-mail it's easy to forget how much time and effort people used to put into letters to family and close friends, and how, over decades, the back-and-forth of correspondence could fill volumes and become a record of one's life and relationships. The fact that letters are personal also conceals the role a regular correspondence can play in sharpening writers' professional talents, encouraging a disciplined approach to writing, developing their powers of observation and reflection, and allowing them to experiment with language. This helps explain how other beloved authors developed late in life.

The Yorkshire veterinarian James Alfred Wight, for example, began writing fiction in the early 1960s, in his late forties, after years of writing diligently to his parents in Glasgow. For nearly a decade, he would spend evenings writing at a portable Olivetti table in the family room. (Between these efforts and his correspondence, it's easy to imagine he put in ten thousand hours of practice as a writer.) After years of rejections, he began to focus on what he knew best: animals, Yorkshire, and the life of a country vet. His first collection of stories was published in 1970, under the pen name James Herriot, as *If Only They Could Talk*. Even as his literary career took off, Wight never gave up his practice, nor did he advertise the book among his clients. As he told his son, a cow didn't care if you were Oscar Wilde. (His mother took to introducing herself as "James Herriot's mother," though.)

Theater manager Bram Stoker produced one of the nineteenth century's most enduring works of fiction while managing the Lyceum Theatre and its owner, the great Shakespearean actor Henry Irving. Stoker joined the Lyceum in 1878, after working as a civil servant and moonlighting as a critic and writer in Dublin. He continued writing on the side. Around 1890, Stoker began work on a story that blended medieval history, Gothic fiction, and the Victorian fascination with the occult and supernatural. He added detail and color from his observations of London's theatrical world and the actors, writers, famous explorers, politicians, and police who made up Irving's social circle. He worked on it during summer vacations in the seaside town of Whitby (the town would become one of the main locations for the story), and then the more remote village of Cruden Bay, in Scotland. Seven years after he began writing it, in 1897, Stoker's *Dracula* was published.

The life of John Ronald Reuel Tolkien, the author of *The Hobbit* and *The Lord of the Rings*, offers the most remarkable example of deep play producing enduring literary work. Tolkien was a professor at Oxford, a father of four, and an excellent scholar. He had an interesting circle of friends: he stood as godfather to John Eccles's first child and was close friends with C. S. Lewis, and the two were members of the Inklings, an informal group of Oxford writers. But little else in his biography foreshadowed his emergence as one of the century's great writers of fantasy. Tolkien's imagination ran deep but for years was private. He had a fascination with languages that began as a child, with his mother's encouragement. Few children would describe themselves captivated by the "surface glitter" of Greek, with its "fluidity . . . punctuated by hardness," or appreciate the feel of the Welsh names on railway cars as they rumbled by a bedroom window, but Tolkien did. He constructed archaic private languages and their modern forms, then created alphabets to match. His mother's death when he was twelve gave the outgoing boy a tragic view of life and fixed in Tolkien's mind an association among his mother, life in the country, and the pursuit of languages. Inventing new languages and imagining the places where they were spoken became a way of keeping her memory alive.

He kept up this private invention for decades. At Oxford, he studied medieval languages and philology, created a new private language based on Finnish (it later evolved into the language of the High Elves in *The Lord of the Rings*), and studied calligraphy both to better decipher old texts and to create new scripts. He began writing modern versions of ancient myths and epics, centered around the fate of three Elven jewels he called the Silmarils. Even after he married, started a family, and undertook scholarly studies of the language of Beowulf and the philology of Middle English, Tolkien continued tinkering with his invented languages and myths. He also began to tell stories to his children. After a few years, he started writing them down. Occasionally he would take ideas—an elf name, a wizard, a place-name—from the myths and weave them into the children's tales. And so, in a slow, almost organic process, *The Hobbit* evolved into an exciting children's story, embroidered with mythical and linguistic details that hinted at a much harder, darker world. Tolkien's stories of Middle-earth are more than imaginative flights or well-told stories. *The Hobbit* and *The Lord of the Rings* are the result of decades of deep play with language, mythology, and storytelling.

The Electric Giraffe is another product of deep play that went in unexpected directions. Lindsay Lawlor isn't a professional animator or robotics expert; he's a fire alarm systems engineer by day. He's been working on fire alarm systems most of his adult life. Working construction after high school, he discovered that "there were so few people who knew about computer equipment who were in the construction industry, if you knew about computers and could do software, you were a god." Installing and maintaining the systems is interesting work: every building is a little different, but every building has to be up to code, and so no two projects are exactly the same. It's also stable. During recessions, businesses will put up with old carpeting and furniture; no one shuts down the fire system.

In other words, it's a good job, and fire alarm systems are essential. But "they're things you'll never use, hidden somewhere you'll never see," he says. "They're noble but boring." Ideally, his systems sit unused and his work remains invisible. The best-made systems "stay as quiet as possible until a true emergency happens." So in a sense you never really know how well you've done your job, and you get little recognition for it. The alarm system job gives Lawlor lots of "windshield time," long periods behind the wheel "when you can let your brain daydream and wander."

The Giraffe offers Lawlor an opportunity to create a technology that's more visible, that has a personality, that people will want to interact with. It also draws on technical skills he developed as a kid. Lawlor grew up in Point Loma, in San Diego, in the 1970s. "I was an only child, and we weren't that rich, so I made my own toys," he recalled. He built lots of model airplanes, laying out patterns, cutting the pieces from sheets of balsa, and gluing them together to form superstructures. He learned how to fix cars and built dune buggies and lawnmower-powered minibikes with his grandfather. "I've been working with structural frames my whole life. There's a lot of knowledge and savvy that comes with that." The Giraffe draws directly on that knowledge. In fact, he says, "the framework in the giraffe is identical to what you'd find in a wooden model airplane." A Japanese toy giraffe robot, which had a central motor that controlled the animal's legs, provided a model for the four legs, which had to be identical because small differences would make for an uneven gait and create stresses on the motor and structure. The rest of the giraffe, though, was an exercise in "free-form welding," guided by Lawlor's inspiration and his experience building models. So the Giraffe is an extension of himself, an expression of his personality, and a project that connects Lawlor to his past.

In conversation, I notice, Lawlor calls the Giraffe "he," never "it." I ask when he began to think of it as a being rather than a machine. "Since day one," he replies. It's always been a "friend, a person, rather than a machine or an art project." Sometimes deep play really does take on a life of its own.

At one point during their games in the Quadrangle Club, Albert Michelson told Norman Maclean, "Billiards is a good game, but billiards is not as good a game as painting, but painting is not as good a game as music, but then music is not as good a game as physics." For Michelson, even if they weren't "as good a game as physics," billiards, painting, and music all offered him a chance to restore his mental batteries, get out of the laboratory, apply his dexterity in pleasing ways, and connect to his childhood and family life in Murphys Camp. They exemplify deep play. Whatever form it takes, deep play provides some of the same challenges and satisfactions as work, at a small scale or more immediate form. It offers a chance to develop additional skills and perspective on life. The choice of activity is often deeply personal and reflects profound personal interests or family history. Deep play is a critical form of deliberate rest and an essential part of the lives of creative people. It provides a way to unify what might otherwise be disparate and scattered activities into a unified whole, a life that is greater than the sum of its parts.

The language that people use to describe deep play offers an important clue to why this process is powerful, and why deep play is so important. There's nothing about mountain climbing that makes it appealing specifically to scientists and no one else. There are also plenty of CEOs and successful doctors, lawyers, and bankers who are mountain climbers, and they often describe the rewards of summiting a peak by reaching for metaphors from their worlds. There are also some world-class climbers who live out of their vans or make just enough money to support their next trip; there are outstanding skiers and surfers who live this way, too. There are also lots of scientists who sail or are passionate amateur musicians or artists, and many of them describe those activities as similar to their work in critical respects.

For creative and prolific people, seeing outside activities as expressions of the same interests that guide their professional lives builds a bridge between the worlds of work and rest and helps turn these activities into deep play. For Michelson and other creative figures, deep play didn't compete with work; it was a way to express the same fascination with nature, need to challenge one's self, and passion for focus and concentration and problem-solving. Seeing them as connected helps turn what could be seen as a time-wasting distraction into an important, valuable part of their lives. It helps justify pursuing these activities even if they're time-consuming.

Deep play is also striking because even if it speaks to the same profound interests and uses common skills, it also establishes clear boundaries between work and play. You may feel that rock climbing is like science, but you can't work on equations while you're hanging thirty feet off the ground. Unlike efforts to achieve work-life balance that end up smearing the two worlds together and lead to your multitasking your way through children's activities, deep play demands exclusive focus.

The ability to see rest and recreation as connected, even as part of a unified whole, was something that Bernice Eiduson and her successors observed in top-performing scientists. As Root-Bernstein put it, elite scientists shared the belief that "time relaxing or engaging in their hobbies could be valuable" to "their scientific efficiency and thus to their careers." For them, playing the piano or painting was just another "expression of a general aesthetic sensibility about nature." What they did in the lab, the court, the climbing wall, and the lecture hall were woven together, different activities linked by common interests and shared passions. Low achievers, in contrast, said nothing about serious hobbies. They "had none or found them irrelevant to their work." Rather than discover the benefits of deep play, the less-accomplished members of Eiduson's cohort assumed that they would do better work by doing more work—and their careers suffered for it.

Finally, it may be that seeing deep connections between work and other activities, and conceiving of activities as deep play, helps creative minds keep working on problems even while playing music or painting or hiking. Seeing mathematics and art as different ways to appreciate the beauty of nature, or hiking as a kind of nature worship, or both mountain climbing and laboratory research as exercises in problem-solving, may make it more likely that your subconscious mind will keep working on problems even as your conscious mind is hitting the trail or breaking camp.

Sabbaticals

I myself had several reasons to start the first sabbatical: One was to fight routine and boredom, another the insight that I could come up with different kinds of projects when given a different time-frame to spend on them. I also expected it would be joyful. What I did not expect was that these sabbaticals would change the trajectory of the studio, and I did not dare to imagine that they would be financially successful. But they were.

—STEFAN SAGMEISTER

EVERY SEVEN YEARS, designer Stefan Sagmeister stops talking to clients, closes up his office, and takes a year off. Born in Austria, Sagmeister worked for advertising agencies in New York and Hong Kong before opening his own studio in 1993. Sagmeister has worked with corporations like Adobe and BMW, museums like the Guggenheim Museum and MoMA, publications like *The New York Times*, and musicians ranging from Lou Reed and Brian Eno to the Rolling Stones and Jay-Z. You can see his intensity in a 1999 poster advertising a lecture in Detroit: it features a picture of Sagmesiter's naked torso with the lecture details carved into his skin. Other pieces are huge, labor-intensive, and one of a kind. An installation in an Amsterdam square spelled out "Obsessions make my life worse and my work better" with two hundred fifty thousand coins, laid out by a hundred volunteers over a week. Another piece was made from ten thousand green and yellow bananas; the green ones spelled "Self-confidence produces fine results." The message disappeared as the bananas aged and blackened.

In 1999, Sagmeister planned his first sabbatical. His firm was doing great, but he was worried that his work was starting to become repetitive. So Sagmeister notified his clients, put some money away, and in 2001 closed up shop. He envisioned all kinds of things going wrong: he would lose his edge, clients would desert him, the design world would leave him behind. When he returned and reopened his studio, Sagmeister was full of ideas: he'd been able to think seriously about design and now, after seven years of constant projects and studio management, had a renewed sense of design as a calling, not just a career or job. Clients came back; if anything, the sabbatical added to his mystique.

Did the sabbatical help his work? Well, in 2005 he won a Grammy, for his design of the Talking Heads box set *Once in Lifetime*, and a National Design Award. After his second sabbatical in 2008–2009, he won another Grammy (for his design of the David Byrne and Brian Eno album *Everything*

That Happens Will Happen Today), and he won the American Institute of Graphic Artists Gold Medal in 2013. His exhibition "The Happy Show," which explores the interface of behavioral science and design, and his own self-experiments on happiness, got its start during his sabbatical. (It represents a major evolution in his thinking, since in Vienna "many embrace misery and think of anything related to happiness as either 'stupid' or 'American,'" he later said.)

Sagmeister's sabbatical year, like his work, pushed the edge of what's possible. Few of us have the creative and commercial confidence, or the financial resources, to take a full year off. But he shows that even in intensely competitive, fast-moving fields, it's both feasible and profitable to take time off to explore deep ideas and, as he puts it, to "try interesting things for which there is normally no space."

Sagmeister isn't the only world-famous artist-entrepreneur who regularly takes sabbaticals to experiment and extend his craft. Spanish chef Ferran Adrià, the father of molecular gastronomy, would close his restaurant for six months each year. Adrià's restaurant, El Bulli, was a world-famous destination among adventurous gourmands in the 1990s. Certainly it was the hardest to get into: it seated fifty people a night (the kitchen staff was almost as large) and eight thousand a season, and more than a *million* people were on its waiting list. Adrià described eating at El Bulli as a theatrical experience, if you imagine an avant-garde production with Björk playing all the roles and costumes designed by Alexander McQueen. Some dishes used foam and frozen vapor to carry taste. Some dishes looked familiar but were made from unexpected ingredients:

a ravioli dish could use calamari rather than pasta, while what looked like caviar would turn out to be honeyed melon. At other times Adrià deconstructed familiar dishes into their component parts: a Spanish omelet would be constituted from potato foam, onion puree, and egg-white sabayon, then served in a sherry glass. Olive oil, a staple of Spanish cuisine, was fashioned into chips and wound into springs. Inevitably, some dishes were more popular than others: the vanishing ravioli made with a Japanese potato and soy film was a crowd favorite, while tea with clams was perhaps more successful as a provocation. In order to stay inventive, Adrià took half the year to play with new ingredients, experiment with new processes, and create new dishes (literally—the restaurant sometimes developed new cutlery, plates, and glasses, and in some instances it was hard to know where the food ended and the dish began). These long sabbaticals have since been imitated in restaurants founded by his former students, and they helped make El Bulli the world's best restaurant until Adrià closed it in 2011—to focus his energy on consulting and conducting research on creativity processes.

"Taking sabbaticals," Sagmeister told a Spanish interviewer in 2014, "was the best business idea and perhaps also the best creative idea I've ever had." His experience shows that even in a hypercompetitive field, a well-designed break from your normal working routine can recharge your creativity, help you discover new ideas, or lead you to achieve a breakthrough in your current work. And this doesn't just apply to artists: scientists, writers, engineers, and even military commanders can benefit from sabbaticals.

What they all teach us is that to stay ahead, it's necessary sometimes to step back. To keep up, it's good sometimes to slow down.

EXECUTIVES AT COMPANIES and nonprofits generally can't afford to spend a year or six months away from the office, but Microsoft cofounder Bill Gates showed how even a single, well-structured week off every year could benefit a leader. When he was CEO and chairman of Microsoft, Gates's week away from the office—as well as from family and friends (from everyone, in fact, save an unobtrusive cook and caretaker)—took place in a small waterfront cottage with a view of the Olympic Mountains, in western Washington. He didn't read Spinoza or science fiction; most of his reading was super technical and dealt with new technologies and proposals for Microsoft projects. The best way to clearly see industry trends, identify new technologies the company should invest in or develop, and become aware of opportunities and dangers, Gates discovered in the 1980s, was to get away from Microsoft for a week. Some "think weeks" were devoted to particular technology areas: in 2004, for example, he focused most of the week immersed in the literature on wireless technologies. During one famous think week in 1995, Gates realized the importance of the Internet to Microsoft's future business; he returned from other think weeks determined to move Microsoft into Web browsers, tablets, and online gaming.

As a result, Gates's think week has since been imitated by executives at Microsoft and a number of Silicon Valley companies. It's not just executives at big companies that take sabbaticals: Michael Karnjanaprakorn, the CEO of New York–based start-up Skillshare, takes a week off twice a year. Others take a long sabbatical after years of building and running a company: Southern California craft-brewing pioneer Greg Koch took six months off after seventeen years as CEO of Stone Brewing, while South African Johann Rupert, founder of luxury goods company Richemont (which owns Cartier, Vacheron Constantin, IWC Schaffhausen, Montblanc, and other companies) took a year's sabbatical. Many CEOs have found that getting away from the pressures of office politics, the thousands of minor decisions they have to make every day, and the cognitive whiplash that comes from jumping from one subject to another every few minutes, gives them a chance to get a broader perspective on their companies and industries. Sabbaticals improve employee satisfaction, give returning workers a greater sense of clarity about their jobs and future, and improve retention levels.

A few farsighted nonprofits and foundations have also started supporting sabbaticals. A 2009 study of nonprofit sabbaticals found that more than a third of people awarded sabbaticals reported a huge improvement in work-life balance, family connection, and physical health. Three-quarters said they were able to "crystallize an existing vision for their organizations or frame a new one," and 87 percent said they had greater confidence on the job after returning. Interestingly, only 13 percent said the sabbatical made them want to change jobs. For smaller and newer nonprofits, having a few months without the founder also gave the board and staff a chance to develop their own rhythm and style of working. This matches the experience of corporations, where sabbaticals give subordinates a chance to serve as acting CEO, test-drive other roles in an organization, or see whether a succession plan is realistic.

Organizations can also benefit from sabbaticals, as the experience of Samsung Electronics shows. In 1990, when it was still struggling to expand outside Korea, Samsung started an overseas sabbatical program for its most promising executives. Every year, two hundred people attended a three-month boot camp heavy on language immersion, meditation, and education in local customs; they then headed off for six months to one of eighty countries, where they learned the local culture, made friends, and essentially played amateur anthropologist; they then spent another six months working on a business-related project of their own design. Within a decade, the experiences of these graduates were contributing to Samsung's dizzying rise as a global brand. Today, graduates of the sabbatical program are among the company's most senior executives, both in Seoul and around the world.

Samsung Electronics' sabbatical program was implemented during a busy time in the company's history, but fallow periods in an organization can offer unexpected opportunities for executives to develop new skills. America's commanding generals during World War II, for example, came of age during the 1920s and 1930s, when a shrunken military, isolationist sentiment, and the leisurely pace of base life in the Pacific and Philippines seemed to offer few opportunities for advancement. Many observers would have bet that a war would be won by commanders who'd served in Guernica, not Manila. Yet the United States entered World War II with some of the ablest leaders in military history. Why did they even exist? Many ambitious young American officers became frustrated with the fact that, as Lucius Clay (a future general and military governor of post–World War II Germany) said, "your only real return from what you did was your own self-satisfaction," and some who stayed focused on their golf and bridge games. But just as Ferran Adrià used his free time to experiment rather than play cards, another cohort used the interwar years to master modern strategic theory, study economics, learn foreign languages, and observe the rising militaries in Japan and Germany.

For example, George C. Marshall, who became chief of staff of the US Army during World War II, began his career as an aide to General John J. Pershing, then worked as a planner in the War Department. He used a posting in China to study Japan's political and military expansion. As assistant commandant at the infantry school in Fort Benning from 1927 to 1932, he modernized infantry training and strategy. After World War I, Dwight Eisenhower used a posting in Panama to study military history, coauthored a guide to American battlefields in Europe, and spent several years in Washington, DC, and the Philippines. Eisenhower's chief of staff, Walter Bedell Smith, studied guerrilla warfare while posted in the Philippines. For George Patton, a variety of staff postings and time at the War College gave him the chance to sharpen his ideas about mechanized warfare and study the use of tanks by the Germans; in the 1930s, when posted to Hawaii, he studied Japanese militarism and the Imperial Army's campaigns in China. Lucius Clay spent four years in Washington managing public works projects, toured the Philippines with Eisenhower and MacArthur, then spent two years overseeing the construction of hundreds of new airports in the United States. Joseph Stilwell became fluent in Mandarin during three tours in China and a posting as military attaché in Beijing—a talent that made him (somewhat to his regret) the obvious choice to serve as Chinese Generalissimo Chiang Kai-shek's chief of staff during World War II.

In other words, the lack of traditional opportunities and combat assignments in a shrunken peacetime army were not a cause for professional despair. Instead, it offered a chance to pause, to dive deep into subjects that they couldn't investigate during busier times, to question how to organize a modern military, and to lay the foundations for a more professional army. The peacetime army lacked what historian Josiah Bunting III calls a "culture of what we may call 'visible busyness,'" and they took advantage of this slower pace to give themselves "leisure to think, to ponder, to write."

SABBATICALS CAN ALSO play a critical but easily overlooked role in one's intellectual development. These don't have to be the scheduled, well-organized sabbaticals that are a prized feature of academic life. Some of the most powerful, life-changing sabbaticals are relatively short.

For example, Douglas Engelbart, the computer pioneer whose work on online collaborative systems yielded the computer mouse, graphical user interfaces, and a host of other innovations, had an epiphany about the power of computers when he was stuck in the Philippines at the end of World War II. Engelbart had trained as a radar operator in the navy. Dropped on the island of Leyte at the end of the war with little to do but wait for orders home, Engelbart found a Red Cross library "in a genuine native hut, up on stilts, with a thatched roof" and bamboo poles. There, he chanced upon a copy of an essay by Vannevar Bush that explained how electronic technologies might one day help researchers keep track of new research, make associations (or trails, as Bush called them) between ideas, and manage the ever-increasing flow of scientific information. Engelbart was captivated. As a radar technician, he was familiar (as few people were in 1945) with the ways screens could extend users' abilities to process and act on information. Now, he saw a novel use for that technology: to augment human intelligence, manage information, and help people respond more intelligently to the world's challenges. It was a vision that Engelbart would pursue for decades and that would yield technologies that would eventually find their way into the hands of billions and shape the way we think about computers.

Wilder Penfield's neurological career was established by two sabbaticals he took as a young doctor. As a surgeon, he wanted to develop better procedures for repairing brain damage, and he dissected the brains of injured animals in an effort to understand how injuries affect the brain. He soon hit a wall. Using the cell-staining techniques he'd learned from Charles Sherrington while at Oxford, he could see neurons, but could barely make out the glial cells that "nourished and supported the neurons," Penfield recalled. Without understanding how injury affected glial cells, he couldn't move forward. Staining techniques developed by Spanish neurologist Santiago Ramón y Cajal's laboratory could reveal glial cells, and so in 1924 Penfield spent six months with in Madrid, learning how to stain brain sections to more clearly see the damage in glial cells. Four years later, Penfield went to Breslau, Germany, to work with neurologist Otfrid Foerster, who had developed surgical techniques for treating veterans with head wounds that had led to epileptic seizures. Foerster had built a substantial collection of damaged brain tissue samples, but nobody had analyzed the samples, giving Penfield a chance to study damaged human brain tissue on an unprecedented scale; when he combined the samples with the case histories of Foerster's patients, Penfield was able to begin mapping the physical foundations of human neurological disorders. The two trips suggested the benefits that could come from a permanent collaboration between neurosurgery and neuroscience—an idea that drove the creation of the Montreal Institute of Neurology and Penfield's research for the rest of his life.

James Lovelock had many of the critical breakthroughs leading to his Gaia hypothesis during sabbaticals and travels. Lovelock famously spent most of his career as an independent scientist, working from a laboratory in the remote village of Bowerchalke, in the southwest of England, but he was a regular visitor to universities and research centers in the United States. It was during a sabbatical at Yale University in 1958 that he perfected the electron capture detector, a device of exquisite sensitivity that helped demonstrate the spread of chlorofluorocarbons (CFCs) in the atmosphere. In 1961, Lovelock started working with NASA on spacecraft instrument design and began traveling regularly to the Jet Propulsion Laboratory in Southern California. JPL scientists were trying to figure out how to design an instrument that could detect the presence of life on Mars. At the time, most scientists wanted to look for specific organic compounds; Lovelock argued that the earth's atmosphere is dynamic and that life-detecting instruments should look for signs of environmental complexity and rapid change. In September 1965, on another visit to JPL, he realized that the earth's atmosphere doesn't sustain life because it is dynamic; the earth's living systems are "regulating the atmosphere and keeping it at its constant composition," allowing themselves to survive and flourish. A few years later, a visit to the National Center for Atmospheric Research in Boulder, Colorado, "enlightened me on just how biological our atmosphere really was," an insight that he expanded over the next fifteen years while working with biologist Lynn Margulis at Boston University and atmospheric scientist Robert Charlson at the University of Washington.

To put the development of the Gaia hypothesis in Graham Wallas's terms, the preparation and incubation may have taken place largely at Lovelock's Bowerchalke home, but the moments of illumination happened while Lovelock exchanged the solitude of village life for the intellectually crowded atmospheres of JPL, Boulder, Boston, and

Washington. Bowerchalke was an escape from the world of small-bore, bureaucratic science, a place where he could reach the state of sustained concentration that Santiago Ramón y Cajal considered essential for creative endeavor; but whenever he traveled to Pasadena, he later recalled, he "felt like young apprenticed artists must have felt" in "the studios of a Leonardo or a Holbein." Lovelock's travels exposed him to new problems and collaborators, quickened his mind, and inspired him to make new connections and creative leaps.

Indeed, this pattern of years of preparation and incubation at home followed by insights on the road is visible in Graham Wallas's own work. Wallas cofounded the London School of Economics in 1895 and spent his career there teaching political science, but it was a trip to the United States in the summer of 1923 that gave him space to explore "the art of thinking." He had touched on the subject in earlier books, but a two-week voyage across the Atlantic gave him the chance to do "a good deal of fresh thinking" and explore connections among psychology, literary criticism, history, and educational theory. A series of lectures at Dartmouth College forced him to organize his ideas and "developed greatly the ideas of [his] book." Wallas would labor on the project for more than two years, but *The Art of Thought* took shape during that trip.

ONE COMMON FEATURE of the travels and sabbaticals of Sagmeister, Engelbart, Penfield, Lovelock, and Wallas is that they mix alien and familiar elements. Sagmeister consciously sought out new locations that could provide stimulation and renewal. Engelbart had time on Leyte to think about the future of computers at a moment when he and his friends could once again contemplate a peaceful future. The direction of Penfield's scientific research was set on journeys to Spain and Germany, where he absorbed the knowledge created at laboratories with very long and robust traditions. Lovelock spent years moving between the quiet village of Bowerchalke and the Oz-like world of NASA and the Jet Propulsion Laboratory. Getting away from the distractions and demands of London and journeying to the "lovely little academic village" of Hanover, New Hampshire, helped Wallas clarify his ideas about the art of thought. But can we say that these kinds of exposures to different environments really make a difference in creative lives?

Arguments about the psychological and creative benefits of traveling, studying, or working abroad are as old as grand tours of Europe. Recently psychologists have been measuring the effects of travel, exposure to new cultures, and experience living abroad on creativity. This work indicates that while merely traveling somewhere doesn't make you a Paul Gauguin or Elizabeth Gilbert, extended exposure to other places and cultures can increase your creativity.

Some of these studies measured creative performance in the laboratory. In one experiment, psychologists found that people who were reminded of times they had to learn about other cultural norms did better on Guilford's Alternative Uses Test than those who weren't primed. Subjects who thought about times they'd learned about the logic behind unfamiliar norms—why it's good manners in China to leave food on your plate, or why some cultures have strict rules about extending hospitality to strangers—did even better. In another experiment, MBA students who moved easily between two different cultures did better on several creativity tests than children of immigrants who either felt like perpetual outsiders or had fully assimilated.

The problem with studying creativity by measuring performance on tests is that it's not clear that laboratory tests measure the same kind of creativity we use in real life. As scientists put it, the small-c creativity demonstrated in experiments may not tell us a lot about the large-C creativity of the real world. To answer these concerns, Columbia Business School professor Adam Galinsky and his collaborators looked at the careers of biculturals, people "who identified with both their home and host cultures." In one study, they tracked the careers of Israeli engineers in Silicon Valley companies and compared the promotion histories and reputations of biculturals to those who had assimilated to American culture and those who felt like aliens. They found that bicultural engineers were promoted faster and had better reputations among their bosses and peers. In an industry that prizes the ability to be innovative, to get inside the minds of your customers, and to spot new opportunities, biculturalism made a measurable difference in who got ahead.

Galinsky and his collaborators at INSEAD studied another industry whose leaders travel regularly, have the opportunity to regularly express their creative vision, and are under constant pressure to innovate: fashion. Top designers circulate between Paris, New York, Milan, and London; they must create new lines of clothes and accessories at least twice a year; and their work is subject to constant scrutiny and critical review. Galinsky and his colleagues collected eleven years' worth of ratings by the French trade magazine *Journal du Textile* of major fashion house lines. (Conveniently, the *Journal* asks buyers—the people who decide which lines will appear in stores—to rate the creativity of a collection on a scale of 0 to 20.) They then looked for relationships between a designer's ratings and their foreign experience. They considered the breadth of experience designers had abroad, measured by how many countries they worked in. They also considered depth, defined by how long designers lived abroad. Finally, they estimated the cultural distance between a designer's home and where they visited.

What they found was that all three factors contributed to increases in a designer's creativity, though the timing of the impacts varied. Breadth and cultural distance gave designers a creative boost early on, but in the long run, depth—how long they spent living abroad—was most important. Learning to adjust to a new place requires going through culture shock, adapting to new surroundings, making new friendships and professional connections, and developing an ability to make sense of unfamiliar norms and customs; that won't happen if you hop from fashion show to fashion show and never leave the world of hotel chains, conference centers, and international airports. However, even a short period working abroad was better than nothing: the worst thing a creative designer could do was play it safe and stay home. They also found that the impact of time abroad was curvilinear:

the benefits would rise, peak, and eventually start to decline, forming an inverted U. In other words, working in two countries in a year was stimulating, but working in seven or eight was overwhelming: you just didn't have time to assimilate or internalize what you'd seen. Likewise, the cultural distance between Milan and New York might be stimulating, but the distance between Milan and Kabul is vast. Navigating the demands of another culture could force you to become more open, set aside old prejudices, and embrace new ideas; but all that energy could also be absorbed in learning a difficult language and dealing with culture shock.

"EVERYONE WHOSE JOB description includes 'thinking' or coming up with ideas will benefit from" taking a sabbatical, Stefan Sagmeister says. His experiences and the sabbaticals of Ferran Adrià, Bill Gates, and the Samsung executives varied greatly in length, regularity, and location, but they all show how well-designed breaks can offer opportunities for creative recovery. As they escaped their everyday environments and were free to pursue high-level goals without the constraints of detailed schedules, their sabbaticals provided opportunities for professional and personal renewal that they could draw on to build their companies and careers. The careers of Douglas Engelbart, Wilder Penfield, and James Lovelock show how sabbaticals can spark life-altering discoveries and epiphanies, and become occasions for transformation rather than restoration. Finally, creative, self-motivated American army officers treated the slack of the interwar era as an opportunity to immerse themselves in military history and strategic theory, study the growth of the Japanese and German militaries, and master languages.

Together, these examples show how being in an environment that is new but not alienating, intellectually stimulating, and different from home helps free the mind to make creative leaps. Sagmeister spent part of his sabbatical in Bali, an island that is at once exotic and accessible to Western visitors. For Gates, a secluded and remote cabin offered a break from the constant demands of the executive suite. Leyte was an American base a world away from Engelbart's home, a place where he could think about how wartime information technologies could be used in the future. Penfield had to navigate unfamiliar cultures in Madrid and Breslau, but Ramón y Cajal's and Foerster's institutes were global centers of neuroscience and neurosurgery: being there broadened his cultural horizons, deepened his already dazzling professional pedigree, and gave him the skills and vision to combine neurosurgery and neuroscientific research. Lovelock moved from the quiet of an English village to American universities and the kinetic environment of NASA at the height of the space race.

Successful sabbaticals are also periods of detachment from one's regular life. Bill Gates's mansion in Medina, Washington, is sixty-six thousand square feet, but his think week cabin doesn't accommodate family or assistants and is only accessible by seaplane. Sagmeister and Adrià closed down their businesses during their breaks and weren't accessible to clients or patrons. (For academics, detachment is an important factor in the success of academic sabbaticals, according to a 2010 comparative study of academics in Israel, New Zealand, and the United States.)

The most fruitful sabbaticals, like other forms of deliberate rest, are active. James Lovelock was energized by his travels and visits with collaborators, just as his deep thinking was sustained by life in Bowerchalke. Penfield worked intensely in Madrid and Breslau, but those sabbaticals were rejuvenating. Gates would read up to eighteen hours a day and sometimes didn't even go outside until Wednesday afternoon. Wallas's trip to the United States combined periods of uninterrupted reflection with an intense schedule of lectures and seminars. It doesn't sound terribly restful, but by now it shouldn't come as a surprise that the right kind of strenuous activity, done under the right circumstances, can be restorative. If even military service can serve as a psychological break from a job, so can a week by a lake with a stack of offprints and technical reports.

Finally, while we usually think of sabbaticals as long (perhaps prohibitively so), they don't have to be. As Adam Galinsky showed, long immersion in other cultures and the development of a bicultural identity have measurable, beneficial effects on the work of people as different as engineers and fashion designers. Yet a weeklong sabbatical can be restorative when done skillfully, and even a monthlong sabbatical can be life-changing.

Conclusion:
The Restful Life

It is neither wealth nor splendor, but tranquility and
occupation, which give happiness.

—Thomas Jefferson

In this book, I've argued that we should treat work and
rest as equals; that we should treat rest as a skill; that the
best, most restorative kinds of rest are active; and that when
practiced well, rest can make us more creative and productive, without forcing us into a funhouse mirror of endless
work and ever-rising expectations. A life that takes rest seriously is not only a more creative life. When we take the right
to rest, when we make rest fulfilling, and when we practice
rest through our days and years, we also make our lives richer
and more fulfilling.

Rest doesn't just magically appear when we need it, especially in today's busy world. Taking rest seriously requires

recognizing its importance, claiming our right to rest, and carving out and defending space for rest in our daily lives. We have to choose to make an earlier start to the day to earn time to rest later; we have to reserve space on the daily calendar for a walk, or keep time free on the weekends for a hobby or sport; we must arrange our finances and business affairs so we can take a sabbatical.

When rest goes from being something that perches in the leftover hours between work and sleep (and housecleaning and child-rearing and volunteering and commuting, and so on, ad infinitum) to being something that you claim for yourself, it becomes more valuable and tangible. As behavioral scientists will tell you, vague plans and ambitions are far less likely to bring success than specific goals. The very act of making specific plans helps make a goal feel more realistic and accessible, and gives you a clearer sense of its value. Deliberate rest is not a negative space defined by the absence of work or something that we hope to get sometime. It is something positive, something worth cultivating in its own right.

Taking rest seriously also helps bring more of your life into clearer focus. At the everyday level, it heightens your ability to concentrate and discourages multitasking. Protecting time for rest also forces you to consider whether a new opportunity, request for a favor, or demand on your time is really worth it. It helps you identify tasks that you might casually accept and regret later, and gives you permission to (diplomatically) turn them down. It helps contain our impulse to be (and to publicly appear to be) super busy and lets us focus on a small number of things that really matter to us, rather than pursue too many things. Too often busyness is not a means to accomplishment but an obstacle to it. Deliberate rest helps you recognize and avoid the trap of pointless busyness and concentrate instead on what's important.

A life that focuses on what matters most, makes time for rest, and declines unnecessary distractions may look simple on the outside, but from the inside it is rich and fulfilling. As the author Annie Dillard put it, "Who would call a day spent reading a good day? But a life spent reading—that is a good life. . . . A day that closely resembles every other day of the past ten or twenty years does not suggest itself as a good one. But who would not call Pasteur's life a good one, or Thomas Mann's?"

So deliberate rest helps organize your life. It also helps calm your life. After spending a weekend at High Elms, Herbert Spencer observed a "remarkable peculiarity" about John Lubbock: his days were full of "many and varied occupations," yet "he never seemed in a hurry." Even when turning his attention to business after a morning spent hunting with his brothers, moving between meetings and his bank, or running off to deliver a lecture, "by his habitual calm, [Lubbock] gave the impression that he was quite at leisure."

Today, we treat being stressed and overworked as a badge of honor, a sign of seriousness and commitment; but this is a recent phenomenon, and it inverts traditional ideas of how leaders and professionals should behave under pressure. For most of history, leaders were supposed to appear calm and unhurried; success began with self-mastery and self-control.

As early as the sixth century BCE (before Plato and Aristotle), Chinese general Sun Tzu wrote in *The Art of War*, "It is the unemotional, reserved, calm, detached warrior who wins, not the hothead seeking vengeance and not the ambitious seeker of fortune." In *The Book of Five Rings*, written around 1645, Japanese swordsman Miyamoto Musashi advised, "Both in fighting and in everyday life you should be determined though calm."

Today's workplace moves us backward, and weakens our spirit. It is a mistake to assume that the most frazzled and panicked workers are the most serious. As William James wrote in "The Gospel of Relaxation," "eagerness, breathlessness, and anxiety are not signs of strength: they are signs of weakness and of bad coordination."

Deliberate rest helps cultivate calm. It deepens your capacity to focus, which helps you complete urgent tasks while driving off anxiety. It encourages you to work steadily rather than wait for a burst of inspiration (or simply the last minute). It reduces the number of things you have to do by helping you recognize and turn down inessential tasks. Finally, it deepens your emotional reserves and resilience, which makes it more likely that you'll meet challenges with greater confidence.

This kind of calm is also valuable in workplaces that expect high levels of emotional engagement. As sociologist William Davies argues, today's workers are told that passion is their greatest asset and that they should do what they love (or at least love what they do); employers, meanwhile, have come to see happiness as a strategic resource that boosts employee productivity, decreases absenteeism and turnover, and increases customer satisfaction. In a few very privileged companies, where competition for talent is ferocious, this translates into free food, entertainment, on-site dry-cleaning, and other perks; elsewhere, it's deployed as a kind of weaponized positive psychology, in which automated systems watch for signs of discontent, negative voice tone during customer phone calls, and indicators that happiness is at suboptimal levels. In environments like these, the ability to detach from a workplace that wants to commoditize your emotional life, and to cultivate a private life rather than succumb to easy alternatives that keep you in the office, is more valuable than ever.

Deliberate rest also gives you more time. At an everyday level, deliberate rest helps you work more effectively. It frees time in your calendar by helping you maintain stricter boundaries between work and rest time, and use your leisure time in more fulfilling ways. By helping you find forms of rest that don't compete with work, deep play and deliberate rest reduce your sense of time pressure.

One of the more remarkable findings in the Eiduson study is that the most successful scientists saw their work and leisure as connected and mutually supportive, and expressed fewer anxieties about time pressure. For the top performers, swimming or hiking didn't compete with their time in their laboratory, and they didn't feel that the time they spent on deliberate rest was stolen from more productive things. They were careful not to spend too much time outdoors or pursuing hobbies, but for them, work and rest were all part of a whole.

Indeed, world-class performers often are more likely to call themselves "lazy" than their less-accomplished peers. This isn't just false modesty. Because they seek out forms of rest that give their conscious minds a break and provide a mental and psychological boost but leave their subconscious minds free to run through ideas, test and reject possibilities, and home in on a solution, their sense of how much time they work and how much time they have at their disposal differs from that of their less-successful colleagues. This is why in Eiduson's study, less well-cited or well-known scientists saw themselves as too time-pressed for hiking or surfing or playing the piano: they had too many commitments, too many obligations, too many demands on their time—and the sad belief that if they just worked a little harder, they could get on top of things.

Finally, deliberate rest helps you live a good life.

The fact that deliberate rest is skilled and active makes it more effective, more energizing and restorative, than passive forms of entertainment. Deliberate rest also serves as a hedge against narrowness and intellectual atrophy. This is why some of the strongest advocates for active rest are people in super busy jobs. Neurosurgeon Wilder Penfield, for example, warned medical students that unless they cultivated other interests, "your specializing will expose you to an insidious disease that can shut you away from all but your occupational associates" and "imprison you in lonely solitude." Penfield's mentor, William Osler, warned that without care, "good men are ruined by success in practice," and that "ever-increasing demands" can leave even the most curious person "worn out, yet not able to rest." It was essential to develop "some intellectual pastime which may serve to keep you in touch with the world of art, of science, or of letters."

Over the course of a life, deliberate rest restores your energy, gives you more time, helps you do more, and helps you focus on doing the things that matter most while avoiding those that don't. It helps you craft a life in which you can discover what challenges you're meant to take on and what hard tasks are most rewarding, and gather the energy and have the time and freedom to face them. It creates a life that's rewarding while it's lived, a life that has purpose and pleasure, work and reward, in equal measure. And that life feels complete and well-spent at the end.

But that end may be a long time coming. We often presume that the most creative people are young and that great artistic works or scientific discoveries or innovative products are inevitably the product of self-sacrifice. Certainly there are plenty of geniuses who die young. But when I tallied up the ages of the figures I discuss here, I was surprised to find that many of them lived well into their eighties and were active almost until the end. If you want to burn out and die young, no one will stop you; but if you want to live to a ripe old age, enjoy that life, and be engaged and active throughout, it seems deliberate rest can help you get there.

In his essay on recreation published in his 1895 book *The Use of Life*, John Lubbock makes a distinction between idleness and leisure: "Leisure is one of the grandest blessings, idleness one of the greatest curses," he argues, and "one is the source of happiness, the other of misery." Rest, he argues, is often mistaken for idleness, but it is not. "To lie sometimes on the grass under the trees on a summer's day," Lubbock wrote, "listening to the murmur of water, or watching the clouds float across the blue sky, is by no means a waste of time." When we treat rest as work's equal and partner, recognize it as a playground for the creative mind and springboard for new ideas, and see it as an activity that we can practice and improve, we elevate rest into something that can help calm our days, organize our lives, give us more time, and help us achieve more while working less. Lubbock was right. Rest is not idleness.

Acknowledgments

THE VERY FIRST CLASS I took in college was HSS GH 56, "Invention and Discovery in the Arts and Sciences." The class was held in the Merrihue Honors Seminar room on the fourth floor of Van Pelt Library at the University of Pennsylvania. The room was reserved for courses offered through the university's Benjamin Franklin Scholars honors program. Out of some miracle or clerical error, I had been elected to BFS as an incoming freshman, and I signed up for the seminar at the suggestion of the program's director, Linda Wiedmann. It met the morning after my eighteenth birthday. I got lost on my way to class and showed up late.

The course was taught by Thomas Parke Hughes, who was the most eminent historian of technology in the world. I knew nothing about his reputation, but I immediately liked him. The son of a history professor myself, I had grown up on college campuses, and in my eyes Tom's combination of gentility and scholarly brilliance made him the archetype of the great professor. He was a fellow Virginian; in fact, I discovered, he was a fellow Richmonder, and we had even attended rival high schools decades apart.

Tom is best remembered for his scholarship on large technological systems, for developing a set of questions and methods for understanding how things like railroads, electric power networks, computers, and the Internet develop. He saw an underlying order in the evolution of technological systems, a path that all systems follow as they move out of the laboratory and conquer the world. In this seminar, though, using a mix of history (Carl Schorske's *Fin-de-Siècle Vienna*), history of art (Peter Gay's *Art and Act)*, and science (Silvano Arieti's *Creativity: The Magic Synthesis*), Tom directed our attention to a more intimate, psychological set of questions: What is the nature of discovery? What are the mechanisms underneath the mystery that is creativity? Are there fundamental differences in the creativity of scientists, engineers, and artists?

I loved the class from the beginning. It introduced me to the psychology of creativity and showed me a way of thinking about creativity, invention, innovation, and the relationship between art and science that was at once dazzlingly broad and rigorous. It was exactly the kind of intellectual experience I imagined having in college, and I started thinking about changing majors from engineering to history of science and technology. The following semester I nearly failed my math and computer science classes. My path was now clear.

We never talked in that course about rest as a critical part of the creative process, but by asking what new insight we can draw by focusing on activities that we tend to overlook, I hope I can add to our understanding of invention and discovery, contribute to the enterprise that Tom introduced me to, and answer some of the big questions that he posed in Merrihue. *Rest*'s subject, its style of argument, and its effort to draw on humanities, history of art and science, and current work in brain science and psychology, are all inspired by HSS GH 56.

The course was also the beginning of the other defining relationship of my college years. Through my years at Penn, the Ben Franklin Scholars program gave me an unusual degree of freedom to pursue my own interests, design my own courses, and make my own mistakes—all opportunities I exploited to the fullest, first as an undergraduate, and then as a graduate student. Linda Wiedmann was a tolerant, often-bemused, and eternally patient and helpful presence throughout. She was the heart of a quirky, brilliant experiment, and encouraged all of us in the program to make the most of it. Given my debt to them, it is fitting that I dedicate this book to Tom and Linda.

Fortunately I also have many other people to thank for making this book possible.

First and foremost is my agent, Zoë Pagnamenta, who, along with Sarah Levitt and Alison Lewis at the Zoë Pagnamenta Agency, offered critical advice about the proposal, championed the book, and helped it find a home.

My editor T. J. Kelleher took up the challenge of *Rest* with enthusiasm and skill. Joel Rickett at Penguin UK also provided valuable advice in the book's early stages. Alison Mackeen was a crucial early advocate for *Rest* and convinced me that I would be a good fit at Basic Books. Together, they helped make this a better book.

For taking the time to sit down for interviews, answer questions, point me to new sources, and talk over my ideas, I'm grateful to Josh Berson, Jeremy Blatter, David Bissell, Michael Bliss, Janet Browne, Felicity Callard, Christine Cavalier, Darlene Cavalier, Michael Corballis, Susan Crane, Jessica de Bloom, Elizabeth Cullen Dunn, Kieran Fox, Tal Golan, Gustav Holmberg, Kate Hunter, Marina Janeiko, Lyn Jeffery, Ben Kazez, Catherine and Steve King, Tapio Koivu, David Lavery, Jon Lay, Lindsay Lawlor, Kristen Marano, Marcus Meurer, Jonny Miller, Valentin Minguez, Jennie Germann Molz, Jeroen Nawijn, Jill Nephew, Kathy Olesko, Marily Oppezzo, Gina Ottoboni, Cody Morris Paris, Mark Patton, Annie Murphy Paul, Jonathan Pochini, Scott Pyne, Mike Roy, Brigid Schulte, Gauti Sigthorsson, Jonathan Smallwood, Thomas Söderqvist, Mads Thimmer, Marc Ventresca, Frenzy van den Berg, and Mary Helen Immordino-Yang.

The librarians and archival staffs at the London School of Economics, Newnham College, Cambridge, and the British Library all helped me locate information about Graham Wallas and Lord Lubbock.

For years, Jessica Riskin and Rosemary Rogers have played a small but absolutely critical role in maintaining my life as a scholar. Without their facilitating access through Stanford University's history and philosophy of science program to the vast world of online scholarly journals, this book would not have been possible. The Menlo Park Public Library has also been an invaluable resource. We tend to think of our local public libraries as places to take our children for storytime or to find the latest potboiler; as a result we underestimate how they can sustain serious intellectual inquiry and enrich the life of the mind. While I rely heavily on the Stanford Library network for access to obscure journal articles, my local library is where I turn for everyday needs.

This is the second book inspired by my time at Microsoft Research Cambridge. Once again, I have Richard Harper to thank for extending the invitation to come to Cambridge and discover the value of sabbaticals and deliberate rest.

Finally, thanks to my family: my children, Elizabeth and Daniel, who put up with being left in California while Mom and Dad ran off to England, and most of all, my wife Heather, who was with me at Clowns of Cambridge when I started thinking about rest and creativity, and remains, as always, the best intellectual companion, and the best spouse, one could ever hope for.

Notes

The Problem of Rest

26   **seven hours every workday taking care of children:** This includes
      two hours of primary childcare (e.g., playing with, reading to,
      cooking for, and chauffeuring kids) and another five of secondary
      childcare (e.g., throwing the kids in the car and doing errands).

29   **polymaths such as James:** This was brilliantly parodied in the
      television show *Parks and Recreation,* in which Tom Haverford
      (played by Aziz Ansari) declares himself a "mogul" in the small
      town of Pawnee, Indiana, after opening four restaurants.

The Science of Rest

35   **that region switched off, and other regions lit up:** Let me break
      the fourth wall and add: I could use the scientific names for these
      regions, but unless you have an MD, the names won't mean any-
      thing, and they're incidental to my point. What matters here is that
      the network exists, and its complexity and performance have cog-
      nitive and psychological implications. More generally, throughout
      this book I try to be sparse in my use of technical terms and avoid
      jargon where possible.

42   **Mind-wandering, it seems, enhances creativity by tapping into
      the DMN:** Given that the DMN fires up in periods when we're
      not engaged in conscious thought or focused on our surround-
      ings, it should come as no surprise that mind-wandering and the

default mode network are associated. Neuroscientists recognized almost immediately that DMN research could help shed light on the neurological foundations of mind-wandering and give researchers a better understanding of what goes on inside our brains when it strikes off in pursuit of its own goals. However, they're not two names for the same phenomenon: for one thing, there's evidence that the wandering mind can pull in areas of the brain outside the DMN. But it's clear that the more we learn about the DMN, the more we're going to understand how mind-wandering works.

Four Hours

56 **On this schedule he wrote nineteen books:** Naturally the question arises: how did Darwin make a living? Thanks to his and his wife's inheritances, combined with some shrewd investments, income from Down House's farmland, and a careful eye on the family ledger, Darwin was able to afford the modest but comfortable life of a country gentleman, which left him free to focus exclusively on his science. "My chief enjoyment and sole employment throughout life has been scientific work," he wrote in his autobiography.

60 **apparently short working hours:** Darwin's four-to-five-hour day has an easy explanation: he was a super genius whose accomplishments speak for themselves. Talent like his can't be explained, nor can it be emulated. But Darwin himself didn't think he was a genius. "I think that I am superior to the common run of men in noticing things which easily escape attention, and in observing them carefully," he wrote in his autobiography, but he didn't claim the brilliance of an Isaac Newton. His "steady and ardent" love of science, he continued, was "much aided by the ambition to be esteemed by my fellow naturalists," a "desire to understand or explain whatever I observed," and "the patience to reflect or ponder for any number of years over any unexplained problem." His methodical habits had "been of not a little use for my particular line of work." Even his notoriously poor health in middle age "saved me from the distractions of society and amusement." Indeed, he concluded, "with such moderate abilities as I possess, it is truly surprising that thus I should have influenced to a considerable extent the beliefs of scientific men on some important points."

65 **as "methodical or orderly" as a "city clerk":** Whether Charley was admiring or contemptuous of his father's habits is unclear, since Charles lamented that his son "has less fixed purpose and energy than I could have supposed possible."

Walk

96 **nine-acre garden roof featuring a half-mile walking path:** Like Osaka's Namba Park, built on the site of a skyscraper, or parks made from abandoned elevated train lines, like the Promenade Plantée in Paris and Manhattan's High Line (and Jerusalem's Railway Park, and Chicago's 606, and São Paulo's grittier Minhocão, a reclaimed section of freeway), the Facebook roof is designed to offer an easy place for people to meet, stroll, or think.

98 **Pyotr Ilyich Tchaikovsky:** "He had read somewhere that, in order to keep in health, a man ought to walk for two hours daily," his brother Modest said, and he "observed this rule with as much conscientiousness and superstition as though some terrible catastrophe would follow should he return five minutes too soon." But a solitary walk in the Russian woods was not a hardship: to the contrary, he said, it was a source of "wonderful, indescribable" pleasure, "not to be compared with any other experience." Even when completely engrossed in work, he maintained this routine: in an 1883 letter, he described his days as consisting of "breakfast, dinner, and the necessary walk."

Nap

111 **He had gotten into the habit of napping:** As Churchill later explained in his memoirs, his counterpart, the elderly First Sea Lord John Fisher, got up between four and five in the morning, and by the afternoon "the formidable energy of the morning [had] gradually declined, and with the shades of night the old Admiral's giant strength was often visibly exhausted." Churchill "altered [his daily] routine somewhat to fit in with that of the First Sea Lord," getting up later in the morning, then taking a nap after lunch. On this new schedule, Churchill found that he could "work continuously till one or two in the morning without feeling in any way fatigued," and he and Fisher now "constituted an almost unsleeping watch throughout the day and night." It's notable that the

young Churchill would accommodate the elderly admiral because his relations with Fisher were often difficult, as both men regarded themselves as strategic geniuses. Their dynamic illustrated "one of Churchill's strengths," as Oxford historian Roy Jenkins put it: "although he wanted to dominate those around him, he wanted to do it over first- and not second-rate people."

111   **It was one of the inflexible rules:** So firm was this rule that, as his valet recalled, "there was always a bed provided for him in the Houses of Parliament" where he would "get his sleep in before an important debate." He went to great lengths to sleep comfortably when he was traveling. His plane was equipped with a custom-built pressure chamber with a shelf for books and brandy, a telephone, and its own air circulation system to remove cigar smoke. It allowed him to "loll comfortably like an outsized pearl within a gigantic oyster shell," and gave him the extra oxygen his doctors insisted he have at high altitudes.

123   **Edgar Allan Poe:** Poe today is regarded as one of America's great literary innovators, a science fiction pioneer (his 1835 space travel story, "Hans Phaall—A Tale," was a favorite of Jules Verne), the inventor of the detective story (with 1841's "The Murders in the Rue Morgue"), and a startlingly good writer of horror and the macabre. His use of images that "arise in the soul . . . upon the very brink of sleep" in his work led some editors to assume that he was an opium addict. Incredibly, while he drank heavily, had a tumultuous and tragic personal life, was expelled from West Point and fired from several jobs because of his erratic behavior, and died under mysterious circumstances at forty, he never seems to have been a serious drug user.

SLEEP

146   **B-2 pilots:** Even though crews could literally spend three days nonstop in the air, the billion-dollar aircraft didn't have sleeping quarters—a great indicator of how little attention the Air Force gave to fatigue management in the 1970s and 1980s, when the plane was being designed. Instead, pilots took turns sleeping in a ten-dollar folding lawn chair from Walmart.

154   **Jack Nicklaus:** "I was hitting them pretty good in the dream," he said, "and all at once I realized I wasn't holding the club the way I've actually been holding it lately. I've been having trouble

collapsing my right arm taking the club head away from the ball, but I was doing it perfectly in my sleep. So when I came to the course yesterday morning I tried it the way I did in my dream and it worked. I shot a 68 yesterday and a 65 today."

RECOVERY

160 **Telegraph Cottage:** Telegraph Cottage remained a small player in the history of World War II. After Eisenhower left London in late 1942, the cottage passed to Eisenhower's chief of staff, Bedell Smith. Smith was a famous workaholic who thought nothing of twelve-hour days, but he appreciated having a hideout from the demands of the war. Other generals used it after Smith left, and when Eisenhower returned to London in March 1944 during the planning of Operation Overlord, the Allied invasion of Europe, he moved back into Telegraph Cottage. In an odd coincidence, after the war the cottage was the home of Gabrielle Keiller, an art collector whose husband, Alexander Keiller, restored the Avebury stone circles after purchasing them from John Lubbock's widow.

163 **surveys conducted in 2008 and 2010:** A larger 2012 survey of more than seven thousand American physicians found that almost 40 percent reported at least one symptom of burnout and that doctors were 50 percent more likely to suffer from burnout than the general population and almost twice as likely to have work-life balance issues. Among neurosurgeons, the burnout rate jumps above 57 percent. (Dedication also explains why some people find imminent retirement stressful.)

169 **scientists have been avid musicians:** A few studies have suggested that musical training strengthens the brain in ways that may help you be a better scientist. Playing a musical instrument requires a blend of skills that are spread across the hemispheres of your brain. Directing your hands, reading sheet music, keeping time, and following a conductor of other musicians require using different parts of your brain, and musical training strengthens interhemispheric cooperation. Recently, neuroscientists found that mathematically gifted high school and college students had better interhemispheric cooperation than students who were average at math. (In fact, higher degrees of connectivity between brain regions appears to correlate with higher IQ, more sociability, and better memory, as well as higher levels of education and income.)

172   **shorter but more frequent vacations:** Indeed, today, people with the freedom and means tend to take shorter, more frequent vacations: a 2015 study of wealthy Americans found that they prefer to take short vacations every two to three months.

EXERCISE

176   **watching their careers unfold over several decades:** Longitudinal studies are one of the great tools of sociology and psychology. They require patience, confidence, and a research style that's both scientific and novelistic. You're writing about people's lives, with all their complexity and unexpected twists and turns. But they can produce unique insights and data that are used and extended by generations of researchers.

185   **as confident on peaks as in the lab:** This side of Franklin's life is left out of James Watson's unsympathetic account of Franklin in *The Double Helix*, which casts her as cold, difficult, and impossible to manage, and which has plenty to say about his and his male friends' athletic pursuits. But even if elements of Watson's portrait are accurate, Franklin's brilliance, experimental acumen, and intolerance for weakness or stupidity would have won her respect among her peers had she been a man. Contrast Franklin to her Cambridge contemporary Ludwig Wittgenstein: they were both from well-connected Jewish families yet exhibited a casual disregard for privilege, were impatient with lazy thinking, and could be socially awkward. But this behavior earned Wittgenstein adoration from his students and a reputation among colleagues as an unparalleled genius.

190   **Alan Turing:** Like many scientist-athletes, Turing disliked gym class and team sports as a child but later discovered a natural athletic talent as a cyclist and a long-distance runner. Turing ran most of his life. He was also an avid cyclist, for both pleasure and transportation. Turing hated to drive but found cycling even long distances was easy: he once bicycled sixty miles to school, and when working at Bletchley Park during World War II (he helped break the German Enigma code and developed Colossus, a pioneering electronic computer), he would bicycle to Bletchley wearing a gas mask to protect him from pollen. After the war he went on cycling vacations in Europe.

Deep Play

203 **played billiards with the elderly Albert Michelson:** Maclean later said of their relationship, "Now I suppose Nobel Prize winners are a dime a dozen, but in those days we had only two in the whole country; he was one of them, and Theodore Roosevelt was the other. I was very touched, as a young boy from Montana, to be trusted with the acquaintanceship of such an outstanding, strange and gifted man. I think my story about him is one of the best things I ever wrote."

205 **Painting was also deep play for Winston Churchill:** While he claims in *Painting as a Pastime* to have never given much thought to painting before taking it up at forty, Churchill grew up in a world in which paintings were everywhere. When Churchill was born at Blenheim Palace, the Marlborough collection included pieces by Rembrandt, Rubens, Claude, Watteau, Van Dyck, Gainsborough, Holbein, Titian, Caravaggio, Tintoretto, Vasari—a veritable history of art since the Renaissance. (Winston's grandfather was the Duke of Marlborough; Winston and his parents visited Blenheim but didn't reside there.)

210 **the "reward, in both activities, is almost continual enlightenment":** There was a long tradition among scientists of informal climbing before Gill. At Cambridge, John Littlewood and Edgar Adrian climbed the walls of Trinity College, while Alan Turing climbed King's College. Physicist Lyman Spitzer, who discovered rock climbing in middle age, was nearly arrested by university police for climbing Cleveland Tower, the highest tower on the Princeton campus.

210 **first American team to climb K2:** Reichardt's achievements as a climber are quite remarkable: K2 is a peak so remote and hard to reach, even the local Balti people never gave it a name. At high altitudes the climbing is harder and more technical than on Everest. The weather is harsher and more unpredictable than Everest's, and summer monsoon snowstorms (yes, it's so high the monsoons turn to snow) can leave only few days of clear weather.

212 ***Mystery of the Mind:*** Not only did *Mystery of the Mind* (Princeton, NJ: Princeton University Press, 1975) take up questions Penfield first encountered sixty years earlier while studying with biology professor E. C. Conklin, the first draft was reviewed by Charles

Hendel, a Princeton classmate of Penfield's who later taught philosophy at McGill and Yale.

226   **farsighted nonprofits and foundations:** The first program to support sabbaticals for nonprofit executives and social activists was the Alston/Bannerman Fellowship Program. Since its creation in 1988, a number of regional foundations—the Los Angeles–based Durfee Foundation, Alaska's Rasmuson Foundation, and the San Francisco Bay Area's O2 Initiative—have followed suit.

Bibliographic Essay

INTRODUCTION

My book *The Distraction Addiction: Getting the Information You Need and the Communication You Want, Without Enraging Your Family, Annoying Your Colleagues, and Destroying Your Soul* (New York: Little, Brown & Company, 2013) was the first product of my sabbatical at Microsoft Research. My initial thinking about rest was stimulated by Virginia Woolf, *A Room of One's Own* (London: Penguin Books, 2004); John Kay, *Obliquity: Why Our Goals Are Best Achieved Indirectly* (London: Profile Books, 2010); James Watson, *The Double Helix: A Personal Account of the Discovery of the Structure of DNA*, introduction by Sylvia Nasar (New York: Touchstone, 2001).

William James's essay "Gospel of Relaxation" is republished in *On Vital Reserves: The Energies of Men; The Gospel of Relaxation* (New York: Henry Holt, 1911); quotes are from 58, 62, 63. Bertie Forbes's "Recreation" appears in his *Keys to Success: Personal Efficiency* (New York: B. C. Forbes, 1918), 222–230, quotes on 223, 225.

Earlier works that touch on the role of rest and reflection in improving productivity and work-life balance include Carl Honoré, *In Praise of Slowness: Challenging the Cult of Speed* (New York: HarperOne, 2004) and *The Slow Fix: Solve Problems, Work Smarter, and Live Better in a World Addicted to Speed* (New York: HarperOne, 2013); Andrew Smart's *Autopilot: The Art and Science of Doing Nothing* (New York: OR Books, 2014); Tony Crabbe, *Busy: How to Thrive in a World of Too Much* (New York: Grand Central, 2014); Greg McKeown's *Essentialism: The Disciplined Pursuit of*

261

Less (New York: Crown Books, 2014); Josh Davis, *Two Awesome Hours* (New York: HarperCollins, 2015); Christine Carter, *The Sweet Spot: How to Find Your Groove at Home and Work* (New York: Ballantine Books, 2015); Cal Newport, *Deep Work: Rules for Focused Success in a Distracted World* (New York: Grand Central, 2016). Pico Iyer's *The Art of Stillness: Adventures of Going Nowhere* (New York: TED Books, 2014) is a thoughtful paean to doing nothing.

The Problem of Rest

Santiago Ramón y Cajal, *Advice for a Young Investigator*, trans. Neely Swanson and Larry W. Swanson (Cambridge, MA: MIT Press, 2004), 36, 33. On Ramón y Cajal, see Wilbur Sprong, "Santiago Ramón y Cajal," *Archives of Neurology and Psychiatry* (1935), 156–162; Laura Otis, "Ramón y Cajal, a Pioneer in Science Fiction," *International Microbiology* 4:3 (2001), 175–178; Benjamin Erlich, "Santiago Ramón y Cajal: Café Chats," *New England Review* 33:1 (2012), 168–182; and Dorothy F. Cannon, *Explorer of the Human Brain: The Life of Santiago Ramón y Cajal* (New York: Henry Schuman, 1949).

See E. P. Thompson, "Time, Work-Discipline, and Industrial Capitalism," *Past and Present* 38 (December 1967), 56–97, for more on the concept of "task-oriented" versus "time-oriented" work.

Robert Owen's New Lanark and his ideal of "eight hours' labour, eight hours' recreation, eight hours' rest" introduced the concept of the eight-hour day: Margaret Cole's *Robert Owen of New Lanark* (London: Batchworth Press, 1953) remains a good introduction. E. P. Thompson's *The Making of the English Working Class* (New York: Vintage, 1966) is still essential reading on the history of modern labor; see also Daniel T. Rodgers, *The Work Ethic in Industrial America: 1850–1920* (Chicago: University of Chicago Press, 2014); and William Andrew Mirola, *Redeeming Time: Protestantism and Chicago's Eight-Hour Movement, 1866–1912* (Chicago: University of Illinois Press, 2015). Two books by Benjamin Kline Hunnicutt, *Work Without End: Abandoning Shorter Hours for the Right to Work* (Philadelphia: Temple University Press, 1988) and *Free Time: The Forgotten American Dream* (Philadelphia: Temple University Press, 2013), focus more specifically on unions and working hours.

Thomas Parke Hughes, *American Genesis: A Century of Invention and Technological Enthusiasm, 1870–1970* (New York: Viking, 1989) and Nikil Saval, *Cubed: A Secret History of the Workplace* (New York: Doubleday, 2014) are of interest on the history of the modern office and factory.

Collaborative space in office design is discussed in Kimberly D. Elsbach and Beth A. Bechky, "It's More than a Desk: Working Smarter Through Leveraged Office Design," *California Management Review* 49:2 (Winter 2007), 80–101; for a more critical perspective, see John Seely Brown and Paul Duguid, *The Social Life of Information* (Cambridge, MA: Harvard Business School Press, 2000).

William James, "Gospel of Relaxation," 63, discusses overwork; see also "Mental Overwork," Singapore *Straits Times* (11 August 1913), 12; Bertie Charles Forbes, *Finance, Business and the Business of Life* (New York: B. C. Forbes, 1915), 318.

Brigid Schulte, *Overwhelmed: Work, Love, and Play When No One Has the Time* (New York: FSG/Sarah Crichton, 2014) shaped my thinking about overwork and the performative aspects of modern office and service work, as did Matthew Crawford, *Shop Class as Soulcraft: An Inquiry into the Value of Work* (New York: Penguin Press, 2009); Stephanie Brown, *Speed: Facing Our Addiction of Fast and Faster—and Overcoming Our Fear of Slowing Down* (New York: Berkeley Books, 2014); William Davies, *The Happiness Industry: How the Government and Big Business Sold Us Well-Being* (London: Verso Books, 2015); and Peter Fleming, *The Mythology of Work: How Capitalism Persists Despite Itself* (London: Pluto Press, 2015). Winner-take-all economics are described in Nassim Taleb, *The Black Swan: The Impact of the Highly Improbable* (New York: Random House, 2008).

Lakshmi Ramarajan and Erin Reid, "Shattering the Myth of Separate Worlds: Negotiating Nonwork Identities at Work," *Academy of Management Review* 38:4 (October 2013), 621–644, describes how consultants justify overwork and perform busyness; see also Erin Reid, "Embracing, Passing, Revealing, and the Ideal Worker Image: How People Navigate Expected and Experienced Professional Identities," *Organizational Science* 26:4 (April 2015), 997–1017, doi: 10.1287/orsc.2015.0975.

Linda A. Bell and Richard B. Freeman, *The Incentive for Working Hard: Explaining Hours Worked Differences in the U.S. and Germany*, NBER Working Paper No. 8051 (December 2000); Alberto Alesina, Edward L. Glaeser, and Bruce Sacerdote, *Work and Leisure in the U.S. and Europe: Why So Different?* NBER Working Paper No. 11278 (April 2005); Valerie Ramey and Neville Francis, *A Century of Work and Leisure*, NBER Working Paper No. 12264 (May 2006); Mark Aguiar and Erik Hurst, *The Increase in Leisure Inequality*, NBER Working Paper No. 13837 (March 2008); Daniel S. Hamermesh and Elena Stancanelli, *Long Workweeks and Strange Hours*, NBER Working Paper No. 20449

(September 2014) explore trends in working hours and leisure in the United States. For a European perspective see Kimberly Fisher and Jonathan Gershuny, *Post-Industrious Society: Why Work Time Will Not Disappear for Our Grandchildren* (Center for Time Use Research, University of Oxford, 2014); Anna S. Burger, *Extreme Working Hours in Western Europe and North America: A New Aspect of Polarization* (London: LSE Europe in Question Discussion Paper Series, 2015).

David Schrank et al., *2015 Urban Mobility Scorecard* (Texas A&M Transportation Institute, 2015) looks at US commuting hours; for the UK, see Trades Union Councils, "Number of Commuters Spending More than Two Hours Travelling to and from Work Up by 72% in Last Decade," 6 November 2015, online at https://www.tuc.org.uk/workplace -issues/work-life-balance/number-commuters-spending-more-two-hours -travelling-and-work-72. On childcare hours, see the Bureau of Labor Statistics' American Time Use Survey, published online at http://www .bls.gov/tus/. For a broader perspective on family duties, see Charles Darrah, James M. Freeman, and Jan English-Lueck, *Busier Than Ever! Why American Families Can't Slow Down* (Stanford, CA: Stanford University Press, 2007).

Josef Pieper, *Leisure: The Basis of Culture*, introduction by T. S. Eliot (New York: Mentor, 1963), quotes from 40, 41, 42, 24, 20; Immanuel Kant quotes are on 26 and 28.

Ramón y Cajal quotes are from *Advice for a Young Investigator*, 32–38.

The Science of Rest

See Bharat B. Biswal, "Resting State fMRI: A Personal History," *NeuroImage* 62 (2012) 938–944, and Marcus E. Raichle, "The Brain's Default Mode Network," *Annual Reviews in Neuroscience* 38 (2015), 433–447, on the discovery of the default mode network. For a broader perspective, see Randy L. Buckner, "The Serendipitous Discovery of the Brain's Default Network," *NeuroImage* 62 (2012) 1137–1145. Blinking and activation of the DMN is discussed in Tamami Nakano et al., "Blink-Related Momentary Activation of the Default Mode Network While Viewing Videos," *Proceedings of the National Academy of Sciences* 110:2 (8 January 2013), 702–706.

See Stephen M. Smith et al., "A Positive-Negative Mode of Population Covariation Links Brain Connectivity, Demographics and Behavior," *Nature Neuroscience* 18:11 (November 2015), 1565–1567; and Andrew E. Reineberg et al., "Resting-State Networks Predict Individual Differences in Common and Specific Aspects of Executive Function," *NeuroImage* 104 (January 2015), 69–78, on resting state functional connectivity.

See Mary Helen Immordino-Yang, Joanna A. Christodoulou, and Vanessa Singh, "Rest Is Not Idleness: Implications of the Brain's Default Mode for Human Development and Education," *Perspectives on Psychological Science* 7:4 (June 2012): 352–364, on DMN and child development; see also Wanqing Li, Xiaoqin Mai, and Chao Liu, "The Default Mode Network and Social Understanding of Others: What Do Brain Connectivity Studies Tell Us," *Frontiers in Human Neuroscience* 8:74 (February 2014), 1–15; Robert P. Spunt, Meghan L. Meyer, and Matthew D. Lieberman, "The Default Mode of Human Brain Function Primes the Intentional Stance," *Journal of Cognitive Neuroscience* 27:6 (June 2015), 1116–1124.

See Valerie Bonnelle et al., "Default Mode Network Connectivity Predicts Sustained Attention Deficits After Traumatic Brain Injury," *Journal of Neuroscience* 31:38 (21 September 2011), 13442–13451, on DMN damage and cognitive impairment; see also C. M. Sylvester et al., "Functional Network Dysfunction in Anxiety and Anxiety Disorders," *Trends in Neurosciences* 35:9 (September 2012), 527–535; Randy Buckner, Jessica Andrews-Hanna, and Daniel Schacter, "The Brain's Default Network: Anatomy, Function, and Relevance to Disease," *Annals of the New York Academy of Sciences* 1124 (March 2008), 1–38; J. D. Rudie et al., "Altered Functional and Structural Brain Network Organization in Autism," *NeuroImage: Clinical* 2 (2013), 79–94. On hyperconnectivity, see Zhigang Qi et al., "Impairment and Compensation Coexist in Amnestic MCI Default Mode Network," *NeuroImage* 50:1 (March 2010), 48–55.

Jonathan Smallwood quotes are from an interview with the author, 28 July 2015. Other important articles of Smallwood's include Jonathan Smallwood and Jessica Andrews-Hanna, "Not All Minds That Wander Are Lost: The Importance of a Balanced Perspective on the Mind-Wandering State," *Frontiers in Psychology* 4:441 (2013), 1–6; Felicity Callard, Jonathan Smallwood, Johannes Golchert, and Daniel S. Margulies, "The Era of the Wandering Mind? Twenty-First Century Research on Self-Generated Mental Activity," *Frontiers in Psychology* 4:891 (December 2013), 1–11; Jonathan Smallwood and Jonathan W. Schooler, "The Science of Mind Wandering: Empirically Navigating the Stream of Consciousness," *Annual Reviews of Psychology* 66 (January 2015), 487–518.

Michael Corballis, *The Wandering Mind: What the Brain Does When You're Not Looking* (Chicago: University of Chicago Press, 2015) provides a good overview of the literature on mind-wandering.

See Benjamin Baird et al., "Inspired by Distraction: Mind Wandering Facilitates Creative Incubation," *Psychological Science* (August 2012), 1–6, for Baird's study of mind-wandering and creativity; see also Tengteng Tan, Hong Zou, Chuansheng Chen, and Jin Luo, "Mind Wandering and the Incubation Effect in Insight Problem Solving," *Creativity Research Journal* 27:4 (2015), 375–382. Ap Dijksterhuis describes his experiments on mind-wandering and creativity in Dijksterhuis, "The Beautiful Powers of Unconscious Thought," *Psychological Science Agenda* 23:10 (October 2009), http://www.apa.org/science/about/psa/2009/10/sci-brief.aspx.

See Ravi Mehta, Rui (Juliet) Zhu, Amar Cheema, "Is Noise Always Bad? Exploring the Effects of Ambient Noise on Creative Cognition," *Journal of Consumer Research* 39:4 (December 2012), 784–799, on noise, music, and cafés; see also Maddie Doyle and Adrian Furnham, "The Distracting Effects of Music on the Cognitive Test Performance of Creative and Non-Creative Individuals," *Thinking Skills and Creativity* 7:1 (April 2012), 1–7

See Paul A. Howard-Jones et al., "Semantic Divergence and Creative Story Generation: An fMRI Investigation," *Cognitive Brain Research* 25:1 (September 2005), 240–250, on creativity and the DMN; see also Naama Mayseless, Ayelet Eran, Simone G. Shamay-Tsoory, "Generating Original Ideas: The Neural Underpinning of Originality," *Neuroimage* 116 (August 2015), 232–239.

See Weiwei Li et al., "Brain Structure and Resting-State Functional Connectivity in University Professors with High Academic Achievement," *Creativity Research Journal* 27:2 (2015), 139–150, on connections between the DMN and skills-heavy regions of the brain; see also Hikaru Takeuchi et al., "The Association Between Resting Functional Connectivity and Creativity," *Cerebral Cortex* 22:12 (December 2012), 2921–2929; Dongtao Wei et al., "Increased Resting Functional Connectivity of the Medial Prefrontal Cortex in Creativity by Means of Cognitive Stimulation," *Cortex* 51 (February 2014), 92–102; Roger E. Beaty et al., "A Functional Connectivity Analysis of the Creative Brain at Rest," *Neuropsychologia* 64 (November 2014), 92–98.

See Naama Mayseless, Judith Aharon-Peretz, and Simone Shamay-Tsoory, "Unleashing Creativity: The Role of Left Temporoparietal Regions in Evaluating and Inhibiting the Generation of Creative Ideas," *Neuropsychologia* 64 (November 2014), 157–168, on studies of the two-stage model of creativity; on paradoxical functional facilitation, see Narinder Kapur, "Paradoxical Functional Facilitation in Brain-Behavior Research: A Critical Review," *Brain* 119 (1996), 1775–1790; Bruce Miller et al., "Functional Correlates of Musical and Visual Ability in Fronto-temporal Dementia," *British Journal of Psychiatry* 176:5 (May 2000), 458–463; Mark Lythgoe et al., "Obsessive, Prolific Artistic Output Following Subarachnoid Hemorrhage," *Neurology* 64 (January 25, 2005), 397–398; and Narinder Kapur, ed., *The Paradoxical Brain* (Cambridge, UK: Cambridge University Press, 2011).

See Keith Sawyer, "The Cognitive Neuroscience of Creativity: A Critical Review," *Creativity Research Journal* 23:2 (2011), 137–154, on the strengths and limits of fMRI, PET, and other imaging tools. On the broader challenges of connecting laboratory research on creativity with creativity in the wild, see Arne Dietrich, "The Cognitive Neuroscience of Creativity," *Psychonomic Bulletin and Review* 11:6 (2004), 1011–1026; Arne Dietrich and Riam Kanso, "A Review of EEG, ERP, and Neuro-imaging Studies of Creativity and Insight," *Psychological Bulletin* 136:5 (September 2010), 822–848; Anna Abraham, "The Promises and Perils of the Neuroscience of Creativity," *Frontiers in Human Neuroscience* 7:246 (June 2013), 1–9. See Eric Jonas and Konrad Kording, "Could a Neuroscientist Understand a Microprocessor?," unpublished paper, *bioRxiv* (26 May 2016), doi.org/10.1101/055624, for a description of efforts to use neuroscience tools and methods to make sense of a computer chip.

Graham Wallas, *The Art of Thought* (London: Jonathan Cape, 1926; repr. Tunbridge Wells: Solis Press, 2014), quotes from 42 (2014 edition). Despite the popularity of the four-stage model of creativity, Wallas himself gets little attention among psychologists; one exception is Eugene Sadler-Smith, "Wallas' Four-Stage Model of the Creative Process: More Than Meets the Eye?" *Creativity Research Journal* 27:4 (2015), 342–352. Wallas's political writing is the subject of Martin J. Wiener, *Between Two Worlds: The Political Thought of Graham Wallas* (Oxford, UK: Clarendon Press, 1971) and Terence H. Qualter, *Graham Wallas and the Great Society* (London: Palgrave Macmillan, 1980); unfortunately, there is no full-length biography of Wallas.

Helmholtz describes his a-ha moments in Hermann von Helmholtz, *Popular Lectures*, (New York: Longmans Green & Co., 1908), 283. Ragnar Granit describes the "living and creative structures" in a 1972 Nobel address, "Discovery and Understanding," reproduced in *Autobiographies by Nobel Laureates in Physiology or Medicine* (January 2009), 1–13. Henri Poincaré discusses illumination in his book *The Foundations of Science: Science and Hypothesis, The Value of Science, Science and Method* (New York: The Science Press, 1913), 389–390.

Four Hours

Recollections of Charles Darwin, handwritten mss., 1882, Cambridge University Library, CUL-DAR112.B9-B23, contains George Darwin's description of his father's mornings. In the vast Darwin literature, the best recent biographies are Adrian Desmond and James Moore, *Darwin: The Life of a Tormented Evolutionist* (New York: W. W. Norton, 1994), and Janet Browne's two-volume *Charles Darwin: Voyaging* (Princeton, NJ: Princeton University Press, 1996) and *Charles Darwin: The Power of Place* (Princeton, NJ: Princeton University Press, 2003). Darwin's correspondence with his sister was Charles Darwin to Susan Elizabeth Darwin, August 4, 1836, in Francis Darwin, ed., *The Life and Letters of Charles Darwin, Including an Autobiographical Chapter*, vol. 1 (London: John Murray, 1887), 237. Darwin listed the pros and cons of marriage, including "loss of time," in a handwritten list reproduced in Charles Darwin, *The Autobiography of Charles Darwin, 1809–1882: With Original Omissions Restored* (London: Collins, 1958), 232; he describes his ambition, desire "to be esteemed," and "moderate abilities" on 141 and 145, and science as his "chief enjoyment" on 115.

The major sources on Lubbock are Mark Patton, *Science, Politics and Business in the Work of Sir John Lubbock: A Man of Universal Mind* (Aldershot, UK: Ashgate, 2007) and the hagiographic but detailed Horace Gordon Hutchinson, *Life of Sir John Lubbock, Lord Avebury* (New York: Macmillan, 1914). Thomas Hay Sweet Escott describes Lubbock's "lounging grace" in *Personal Forces of the Period* (London: Hurst and Blackett, 1898), 247. Darwin's wonder at Lubbock's productivity is recounted in Ursula Grant Duff, ed., *The Life-Work of Lord Avebury (Sir John Lubbock) 1834–1913* (London: Watts & Co., 1924), 26. Hutchinson describes Lubbock's "prolific," "earnest," and "successful" career on 112, elementary school on 10, ability to switch attention on 32, and enthusiasm for cricket on 27.

Jeremy Gray, *Henri Poincaré: A Scientific Biography* (Princeton, NJ: Princeton University Press, 2013) and Michael Fitzgerald and Ioan James, *Mind of the Mathematician* (Baltimore, MD: Johns Hopkins University Press, 2007), esp. 120, describe Henri Poincaré's working hours. Eric Bell describes Poincaré in Bell, *Men of Mathematics* (New York: Dover, 1937). G. H. Hardy's hours are described in Hardy, *A Mathematician's Apology* (Cambridge, UK: Cambridge University Press, 1967) (see esp. the preface by C. P. Snow and his account of Hardy quoted on 31–32). On Littlewood's schedule, see John E. Littlewood, *A Mathematician's Miscellany*

(London: Methuen and Company Ltd., 1953), and "The Mathematician's Art of Work," *The Mathematical Intelligencer* 1:2 (June 1978), 112–119, quote from 116–117; on Halmos's schedule, see John Ewing and F. W. Gehring, eds., *Paul Halmos: Celebrating Fifty Years of Mathematics* (New York: Springer-Verlag, 1991), and John Ewing, "Paul Halmos: In His Own Words," *Notices of the American Mathematical Society* 54:9 (October 2007), 1136–1144, quote from 1140.

Raymond Van Zelst and Willard Kerr, "Some Correlates of Scientific and Technical Productivity," *Journal of Abnormal and Social Psychology* 46:4 (October 1951), 470–475, describes the Illinois Institute of Technology study; there is also a brief follow-up, Van Zelst and Kerr, "A Further Note on Some Correlates of Scientific and Technical Productivity," *Journal of Abnormal and Social Psychology* 47:1 (January 1952), 129.

Frederic Morton, "A Talk with Thomas Mann at 80," *New York Times* (5 June 1955), online at http://www.nytimes.com/books/97/09/21/reviews/mann-talk.html, describes Thomas Mann's day. The great source on Anthony Trollope is Trollope, *An Autobiography* (London: Blackwood, 1883), quote on 154. On Dickens, see Shelton Mackenzie, *Life of Charles Dickens* (Philadelphia: B. Peterson and Brothers, 1870), esp. 297–300, and John Forster, *The Life of Charles Dickens* (Boston: James Osgood & Co., 1875). His son Charley described his father as a "city clerk" in his habits, as quoted in Mason Currey's *Daily Rituals: How Artists Work* (New York: A. A. Knopf, 2013), 161. On Dickens's attitude to Charley, see Robert Gottlieb, *Great Expectations: The Sons and Daughters of Charles Dickens* (New York : Farrar, Straus and Giroux, 2012), 37.

Many accounts of writers' schedules come from interviews in *Paris Review*, which are available on the *Paris Review* website: Charlotte El Shabrawy, "Naguib Mahfouz, The Art of Fiction No. 129," *Paris Review* 123 (Summer 1992); Jeanne McCulloch and Mona Simpson, "Alice Munro, The Art of Fiction No. 137," *Paris Review* 131 (Summer 1994); Radhika Jones, "Peter Carey, The Art of Fiction No. 188," *Paris Review* 177 (Summer 2006); Peter H. Stone, "Gabriel García Márquez, The Art of Fiction No. 69," *Paris Review* 82 (Winter 1981); George Plimpton, "Ernest Hemingway, The Art of Fiction No. 21," *Paris Review* 18 (Spring 1958); Shusha Guppy, "Edna O'Brien, The Art of Fiction No. 82," *Paris Review* 92 (Summer 1984); George Plimpton, "John le Carré, The Art of Fiction No. 149," *Paris Review* 143 (Summer 1997); Stephen Becker, "Patrick O'Brian, The Art of Fiction No. 142," *Paris Review* 135 (Summer 1995); Thomas Frick, "J. G. Ballard, The Art of Fiction No. 85," *Paris Review* 94 (Winter 1984).

The W. Somerset Maugham quote is related by Hollywood screen-writer Garson Kanin to Pat McGilligan in McGilligan, ed., *Backstory 2: Interviews with Screenwriters of the 1940s and 1950s* (Berkeley, CA: University of California Press, 1991), quote on 104. Saul Bellow's writing schedule is described in Zachary Leader, *The Life of Saul Bellow: To Fame and Fortune, 1915–1964* (New York: A. A. Knopf, 2015), 421–422.

Laura Schellhardt describes writers' schedules in *Screenwriting for Dummies*, 2nd ed. (Boston: John Wiley, 2008), quote on 323; Syd Field's and Robert Towne's daily schedules are described in Syd Field's classic *Screenplay: The Foundations of Screenwriting* (New York: Delta, 2005), quote on 240–241. Scott Adams describes his routine in Adams, "Why 'Dilbert' Creator Scott Adams Wakes Up at 5 a.m. to Do His Most Creative Work," *Business Insider* (24 March 2015), online at http://www.businessinsider.com/the-creator-of-dilberts-morning-routine-2015-3. Stephen King talks about writing schedules (and much more besides) in his *On Writing: A Memoir of the Craft* (New York: Scribner, rep. 2010), quote on 150. Norman Maclean discusses his routine in Nick O'Connell, "Haunted by Waters: A Talk with Norman Maclean," *The Writer's Workshop Review* (28 March 2009), online at http://www.the writersworkshopreview.net/article.cgi?article_id=14; Ingmar Bergman's routine is described in Joe Fassler, "What Great Artists Need: Solitude," *The Atlantic* (4 February 2014), online at http://www.theatlantic.com /entertainment/archive/2014/02/what-great-artists-need-solitude /283585/; on Halldór Laxness, see Peter Hallberg, *Halldór Laxness* (New York: Twayne Publishers, 1971). On the Center for Advanced Study in the Behavioral Sciences, see Tity de Vries, "A Year at the Center: Experiences and Effects of the First International Group of Fellows at the Center for Advanced Study in the Behavioral Sciences, Palo Alto, CA, 1954–1955," in Alasdair MacDonald and Arend Huussen, eds., *Scholarly Environments: Centres of Learning and Institutional Contexts, 1560–1960* (Dudley, MA: Peeters, 2004), 169–180. Arthur Koestler's life is covered in the admirable but not admiring biography by Michael Scammell, *Koestler: The Literary and Political Odyssey of a Twentieth-Century Skeptic* (New York: Random House, 2009).

Thomas Jefferson's account of the "great inequality" is from Willard Sterne Randall, *Thomas Jefferson: A Life* (New York: Henry Holt, 1993), quote on 56. His legal studies are the subject of Davison M. Douglas, "The Jeffersonian Vision of Legal Education," *William & Mary Faculty Publications* Paper 119 (2001), 185–219, quote on 201. His teacher George Wythe also trained Supreme Court justice John Marshal, president James

Monroe, and senator Henry Clay: see Thomas Hunter, "The Teachings of George Wythe," in Steve Sheppard, ed., *The History of Legal Education in the United States: Commentaries and Primary Sources* (Pasadena, CA: Salem Press, 1999), 138–168. Osler describes his hours in his *A Way of Life: An Address to Yale Students, Sunday Evening, April 20th, 1913* (London: Constable and Co., 1913), 50.

Frederick Arnold, *Oxford and Cambridge: Their Colleges, Memories and Associations* (London: The Religious Tract Society, 1873), 375, and Karl Breul, *Students' Life and Work in the University of Cambridge* (London: Bowes and Bowes, 1928), 45–46, are the source of the quotes about reading parties. Useful contemporary accounts include Angelina Gushington, "A Reading Party," in *The Light Blue: A Cambridge University Magazine*, volume 1 (Cambridge, UK: Rivingtons, 1866); Frederic Edward Weatherly [A Resident M.A.], *Oxford Days; or, How Ross Got His Degree* (London: Sampson Low, Marston, Searle & Rivington, 1879); C. W. Ridley, "The Long," in E. W. Badger, ed., *The Cross and Martlets* (Birmingham, UK: Herald Printing Office, 1881); "A Cambridge Man," in *A Guide to the English Lake District, Intended Principally for the Use of Pedestrians* (London: Simpkin, Marshall & Co., n.d.).

Karl Anders Ericsson, Ralf Krampe, and Clemens Tesch-Römer, "The Role of Deliberate Practice in the Acquisition of Expert Performance," *Psychological Review* 100:3 (1993), 363–406, quotes on 390–391, 369, 391; the final quote on the "ability to sustain the concentration necessary for deliberate practice" is from Ericsson, "Attaining Excellence Through Deliberate Practice: Insights from the Study of Expert Performance," in Michel Ferrari, ed., *The Pursuit of Excellence Through Education* (London: Routledge, 2001), 21–56, quote on 29. For an updated perspective on the literature on deliberate practice, see Ericsson and Robert Pool, *Peak: Secrets from the New Science of Expertise* (Boston: Houghton Mifflin Harcourt, 2016); Ericsson, "Why Expert Performance Is Special and Cannot be Extrapolated from Studies of Performance in the General Population: A Response to Criticisms," *Intelligence* 45 (July–August 2014), 81–103; and Scott Barry Kaufman, "A Proposed Integration of the Expert Performance and Individual Differences Approaches to the Study of Elite Performance," *Frontiers in Psychology* 5:707 (July 2014). Malcolm Gladwell uses Ericsson's work in *Outliers: The Story of Success* (New York: Little, Brown and Co., 2008).

Ray Bradbury describes his ten-year apprenticeship in *Zen in the Art of Writing* (Santa Barbara, CA: Joshua Odell Editions, 1994), quote on 62. Carl Emil Seashore discusses the importance of rest in musical training in his *The Psychology of Music* (New York: McGraw-Hill, 1938), quotes on 154–155.

MORNING ROUTINE

The epigraph is from Thomas Mitchell, *Essays on Life* (Glasgow, UK: Vagabond Voices, 2014), 60.

Scott Adams's quotes are from Adams, "Why 'Dilbert' Creator Scott Adams Wakes Up at 5 a.m. to Do His Most Creative Work," and Jessica Zack, "Scott Adams, *Dilbert* Creator, Finds Success in His Failures," *SF Gate* (18 January 2014), online at http://www.sfgate.com/art /article/Scott-Adams-Dilbert-creator-finds-success-in-5156258.php. Adams also describes his morning routine in George Gendron, "Dilbert Fired! Starts New Biz," *Inc.* (1 July 1996), online at http://www .inc.com/magazine/19960701/1721.html; Scott Adams, "How to Make a Comic Strip," *Dilbert Blog* (20 June 2007), http://dilbertblog.typepad .com/the_dilbert_blog/2007/06/how_to_make_a_c.html; Scott Adams, "Diary of a Cartoonist: Dilbert Creator Scott Adams," *Wall Street Journal* (2 May 2014), online at http://www.wsj.com/articles/SB10001424 052702304393704579531732604491594; Vivian Giang, "Dilbert Creator Scott Adams on Why Big Goals Are for Losers," *Fast Company* (14 May 2014), online at http://www.fastcompany.com/3030518/bottom-line /dilbert-creator-scott-adams-on-why-big-goals-are-for-losers.

There's a virtual cottage industry of authors turning out pieces on the morning schedules of CEOs. The 2014 *Quartz Global Executives Survey*, online at http://insights.qz.com/ges/, provides information on the routines and habits of 940 executives, including their morning news-reading habits. My information on Cook, Gross, Dorsey, Schultz, Burns, and van Paasschen is from Max Nisen, Gus Lubin, and Aaron Taube, "22 Executives Who Wake Up Really Early," *Business Insider* (27 August 2014), online at http://www.businessinsider.com/executives-who-wake -up-early-2014-8; Vestberg is interviewed in Tim Dowling, Laura Barnett, and Patrick Kingsley, "What Time Do Top CEOs Wake Up?," *The Guardian* (1 April 2013), online at http://www.theguardian.com /money/2013/apr/01/what-time-ceos-start-day. Laura Vanderkam's *What the Most Successful People Do Before Breakfast* (New York: Portfolio Penguin, 2013) offers a more thoughtful examination of the importance of morning routines.

For a good overview of the mornings of artists and writers, see Mason Currey's *Daily Rituals: How Artists Work*. Currey is the source for my accounts of Frank Lloyd Wright (pp. 131–132) and John Cheever (pp. 110–112); on Wright, see also Maria Stone in Edgar Tafel, ed., *Frank Lloyd Wright: Recollections by Those Who Knew Him* (Mineola, NY: Dover Publications, 2001), 56–62. On John le Carré's morning, see George Plimpton, "John le Carré, The Art of Fiction No. 149," *Paris Review* 143 (Summer 1997); on Hemingway, George Plimpton, "Ernest Hemingway, The Art of Fiction No. 21," *Paris Review* 18 (Spring 1958); Trollope, *An Autobiography*, quote on 153–154; Maya Angelou, quoted in George Plimpton, "Maya Angelou, The Art of Fiction No. 119," *Paris Review* 116 (Fall 1990); on Paul Cézanne, see Walter Pach, "Cézanne—An Introduction," *Scribner's Magazine* 44:1 (July 1908), 765–768, and Émile Bernard, "Memories of Paul Cezanne," in P. Michael Doran, ed., *Conversations with Cézanne* (Berkeley: University of California Press, 2001); Gabriel García Márquez is quoted in Peter H. Stone, "Gabriel García Márquez, The Art of Fiction No. 69."

Psychologists have also studied scheduling, procrastination, and writers. A good introduction is Ronald T. Kellogg, *Psychology of Writing* (Oxford, UK: Oxford University Press, 1999); Ronald T. Kellogg, "Writing Method and Productivity of Science and Engineering Faculty," *Research in Higher Education* 25:2 (1986), 147–163.

Arnold Sommerfeld's advice is related by Werner Heisenberg in an oral history for the Archives for the History of Quantum Physics project conducted by Thomas Kuhn, 11 February 1963, online at https://www.aip .org/history-programs/niels-bohr-library/oral-histories/4661-3. Hans Selye's schedule is described in Hans Selye, *The Stress of My Life: A Scientist's Memoirs* (New York: Van Nostrand Reinhold, 1979), quote on 199. Edna O'Brien is quoted in Shusha Guppy, "Edna O'Brien, The Art of Fiction No. 82," *Paris Review* 92 (Summer 1984); Mario Vargas Llosa is quoted in Susannah Hunnewell and Ricardo Augusto Setti, "Mario Vargas Llosa, The Art of Fiction No. 120," *Paris Review* 116 (Fall 1990).

Mareike B. Wieth and Rose T. Zacks, "Time of Day Effects on Problem Solving: When the Non-Optimal Is Optimal," *Thinking & Reasoning* 17:4 (2011), 387–401, and Cynthia P. May, "Synchrony Effects in Cognition: The Costs and a Benefit," *Psychonomic Bulletin & Review* 6:1 (March 1999), 142–147, are both studies of inhibition and circadian rhythms. See also Christina Schmidt et al., "A Time to Think: Circadian Rhythms in Human Cognition," *Cognitive Neuropsychology* 24:7 (2007), 755–789.

On Alice Munro, see McCulloch and Simpson, "Alice Munro, The Art of Fiction No. 137," *Paris Review* 131 (Summer 1994); on John

Gribbin, see Shelley Kronzek, "Author Interview: John Gribbin," *The Dover Math and Science Newsletter* (21 May 2012), online at http://www.doverpublications.com/mathsci/0521/news.html; on David McCullough, see Elizabeth Gaffney and Benjamin Ryder Howe, "David McCullough, The Art of Biography No. 2," *Paris Review* 152 (Fall 1999).

Isaac Bashevis Singer is quoted in Harold Flender, "Isaac Bashevis Singer, The Art of Fiction No. 42," *Paris Review* 44 (Fall 1968); Toni Morrison's description of her morning and routine is in Elissa Schappell with Claudia Brodsky Lacour, "Toni Morrison, The Art of Fiction No. 134," *Paris Review* 128 (Fall 1993); John Littlewood, "The Mathematician's Art of Work," 116; Stephen King, *On Writing*, 157. Tobias Wolff is quoted in Jack Livings, "Tobias Wolff, The Art of Fiction No. 183," *Paris Review* 171 (Fall 2004); Osler's quote is from his *A Way of Life*, 50; Osler's fellow student Edward Rogers is quoted in Michael Bliss, *William Osler: A Life in Medicine* (Toronto: University of Toronto Press, 1999), 94.

Trollope talks about writing and the question of inspiration in his *An Autobiography*, 72; Raymond Chandler to Alex Barris, March 18, 1949, reproduced in Raymond Chandler with Dorothy Gardiner and Katherine Sorley Walker, *Raymond Chandler Speaking* (Berkeley, CA: University of California Press, 1997), 79–80; Bergman is quoted in Fassler, "What Great Artists Need: Solitude"; Tchaikovsky is quoted in Vera John-Steiner, *Notebooks of the Mind: Explorations of Thinking* (Oxford, UK: Oxford University Press, 1997), 73; Joyce Carol Oates is quoted in Robert Phillips, "Joyce Carol Oates, The Art of Fiction No. 72," *Paris Review* 74 (Fall–Winter 1978); King, *On Writing*, 156–157.

See Sandra Ohly, Sabine Sonnentag, and Franziska Pluntke, "Routinization, Work Characteristics and Their Relationships with Creative and Proactive Behaviors," *Journal of Organizational Behavior* 27 (2006), 257–279, and Lucy L. Gilson, John E. Mathieu, Christina E. Shalley, and Thomas M. Ruddy, "Creativity and Standardization: Complementary or Conflicting Drivers of Team Effectiveness?" *Academy of Management Journal* 48:3 (June 2005), 521–531, on routine and creativity. On the chef's mise-en-place, see Leslie Brenner, *The Fourth Star: Dispatches from Inside Daniel Boulud's Celebrated New York Restaurant* (New York: Clarkson Potter, 2002); Alan Gelb and Karen Levine, *A Survival Guide for Culinary Professionals* (Clifton Park, NY: Delmar Cengage Learning, 2004); and especially Michael Ruhlman, *The Making of a Chef: Mastering Heat at the Culinary Institute of America* (New York: Macmillan, 2009).

Concluding section quotations are from Stephen King, *On Writing*, 157; Henri Poincaré, *Foundations of Science*, 389; the Pablo Picasso quote is widely cited, but its original source is not clear; Chuck Close is quoted in Chris Orwig, *The Creative Fight: Create Your Best Work and Live the Life You Imagine* (San Francisco: Peachpit Press, 2015); a slightly different version of the quote appears in Christopher Finch, *Chuck Close: Life* (New York: Prestel Verlag, 2010), chapter 25; Anthony Trollope, *My Autobiography*, 153.

WALK

The famous Kierkegaard quote about walking comes from a letter from Kierkegaard to his sister-in-law Henriette Kierkegaard, reproduced in Søren Kierkegaard, *The Essential Kierkegaard* (Princeton, NJ: Princeton University Press, 2013), 502. On the history of walking and its philosophical dimension, see Rebecca Solnit, *Wanderlust: A History of Walking* (New York: Penguin, 2000); Geoff Nicholson, *The Lost Art of Walking* (New York: Riverhead Books, 2008).

The Thomas Jefferson quote is from Jefferson to Peter Carr, 19 August 1785, republished on the Monticello website at http://www .monticello.org/site/research-and-collections/exercise; C. S. Lewis describes his walks in *Surprised by Joy: The Shape of My Early Life* (New York: Harcourt Brace, 1984), 142; Graham Wallas's walking is documented in correspondence between himself and his wife, in the Wallas Family Papers, Newnham College, Cambridge; Alice Munro is quoted in McCulloch and Simpson, "Alice Munro, The Art of Fiction No. 137," *Paris Review* 131 (Summer 1994); the Dickens quote is from Forster, *Life of Charles Dickens*, 218; Travis Kalanick's walks are described in Maya Kosoff, "Travis Kalanick Says He Walks 40 Miles a Week Inside Uber's San Francisco Headquarters," *Business Insider* (8 September 2015), online at http://www.businessinsider.com/uber-ceo-travis-kalanick-walks -40-miles-a-week-in-his-office-2015–9; Tony Schwartz discusses energy management in Tony Schwartz and Catherine McCarthy, "Manage Your Energy, Not Your Time," *Harvard Business Review* (October 2007), online at https://hbr.org/2007/10/manage-your-energy-not-your-time.

David Haimes, "An Update on Walking Meetings," *David Haimes* (blog) (24 January 2014), online at https://davidhaimes.wordpress.com /2014/01/24/an-update-on-walking-meetings/, is the source of the quote about writing code and walking meetings. Russell Clayton, Chris Thomas, and Jack Smothers, "How to Do Walking Meetings Right," *Harvard Business Review* (August 2015), online at https://hbr.org/2015/08 /how-to-do-walking-meetings-right, discusses walking meetings among

managers; Silicon Valley walking meetings are covered in Margaret Ta-
lev and Carol Hymowitz, "Zuckerberg, Obama Channel Jobs in Search
for Alone Time," *Bloomberg* (29 April 2014), online at http://www
.bloomberg.com/news/2014–04–30/walking-is-the-new-sitting-for
-decision-makers.html; Craig Dowden, "Steve Jobs Was Right About
Walking," *Financial Post* (12 December 2014), online at http://business.
financialpost.com/executive/strategy/steve-jobs-was-right-about-walking;
Jay Yarow, "When Mark Zuckerberg Really Wants to Hire You, He'll
Ask You to Take a Walk with Him in the Woods," *Business Insider* (7 July
2011), online at http://www.businessinsider.com/mark-zuckerberg-walk
-in-the-woods-2011–7; on Ted Eytan's advocacy of walks, see Alina Dizik,
"Forget Standing Meetings, Try This Instead," *BBC Capital* (5 May 2015),
online at http://www.bbc.com/capital/story/20150504-to-cure-meeting
-mayhem-try-this; Jeff Weiner describes his walking meetings in "Where
I Work: I'll Take Walking 1:1s Over Office Meetings Any Day," *LinkedIn
Pulse* (29 January 2013), online at https://www.linkedin.com/pulse
/20130129033750–22330283-where-i-work-i-ll-take-walking-1–1s-over
-office-meetings-any-day; Florey and Chain's walks are described in E. P.
Abraham, "Howard Walter Florey, Baron Florey of Adelaide and Marston, 1898–1968," *Biographical Memoirs of Fellows of the Royal Society* 17
(November 1971), 255–302.

Katherine Simon Frank, "Herbert A. Simon: A Family Memory,"
online at http://www.cs.cmu.edu/simon/kfrank.html, discusses walking
and loosening creative inhibitions; Watson and Crick's walks are described in Watson, *The Double Helix*. Richard Thaler describes his walks
with Kahneman and Tversky in his memoir, *Misbehaving: The Making of
Behavioral Economics* (New York: W. W. Norton, 2015). Tchaikovsky's
walks are described by his brother in Modest Ilich Tchaikovsky, *The
Life and Letters of Peter Ilich Tchaikovsky* (New York: John Lane, 1906),
quotes on 491, 263, 447; on Ludwig van Beethoven's walks in Vienna,
see Anton Schindler, *The Life of Beethoven* (Boston: Oliver Diston, 1900).
Lin-Manuel Miranda talks about his walks in Patrick Healy, "Walking
the Dog to Awaken the Muse," *New York Times* (21 March 2014), MB2;
Suzy Evans, "How 'Hamilton' Found Its Groove," *American Theatre* (27
July 2015), http://www.americantheatre.org/2015/07/27/how-hamilton
-found-its-groove/; Rebecca Milzoff, "Lin-Manuel Miranda on Jay Z, 'The
West Wing,' and 18 More Things That Influenced 'Hamilton,'" *Vulture*
(29 July 2015), http://www.vulture.com/2015/07/lin-manuel-mirandas
-20-hamilton-influences.html.

Eugene Paul Wigner, *The Recollections of Eugene P. Wigner as Told to Andrew Szanton* (New York: Plenum Press, 1992), 228; Paul Dirac, interview with Thomas Kuhn and Eugene Wigner, 1 April 1962, Niels Bohr Library and Archives, American Institute of Physics, https://www.aip.org/history-programs/niels-bohr-library/oral-histories/4575–1.

See Peter Aspinall, Panagiotis Mavros, Richard Coyne, and Jenny Roe, "The Urban Brain: Analysing Outdoor Physical Activity with Mobile EEG," *British Journal of Sports Medicine* 49:4 (March 2015), 1–6, on walking in different environments. On the restorative value of natural environments, see Stephen Kaplan, "The Restorative Benefits of Nature: Toward an Integrative Framework," *Journal of Environmental Psychology* 16 (1995): 169–182.

Nathaniel C. Comfort, *Tangled Field: Barbara McClintock's Search for the Patterns of Genetic Control* (Cambridge, MA: Harvard University Press, 2001), quote on 68, includes McClintock's description of her time at Stanford. Hamilton's walking is described in Robert Graves, *Life of Sir William Rowan Hamilton*, 2 vols. (Dublin, UK: Hodges, Figgis, and Co., 1882); quote is from Hamilton to Rev. Archibald H. Hamilton, August 5, 1865, online at http://www.maths.tcd.ie/pub/HistMath/People/Hamilton/Letters/BroomeBridge.html. Heisenberg's struggle to articulate the uncertainty principle and his walk in Fælland Park are in John Gribbin, *Erwin Schrodinger and the Quantum Revolution* (New York: Wiley, 2013); Heisenberg, interview with Thomas Kuhn and John Heilbron, 5 July 1963, Niels Bohr Library and Archives, American Institute of Physics, online at https://www.aip.org/history-programs/niels-bohr-library/oral-histories/4661–11. Ernö Rubik is quoted in Dave Simpson, "Erno Rubik: How We Made Rubik's Cube," *The Guardian* (26 May 2015), online at https://www.theguardian.com/culture/2015/may/26/erno-rubik-how-we-made-rubiks-cube; see also Noah Davis, "How Ernö Rubik Created the Rubik's Cube," *Mental Floss* (August 2014), http://mentalfloss.com/article/58162/how-erno-rubik-created-rubiks-cube; George Webster, "The Little Cube That Changed the World," *CNN* (11 October 2012), http://www.cnn.com/2012/10/10/tech/rubiks-cube-inventor/.

Interview with Marily Oppezzo, 6 August 2015 at Stanford, is the source of the quotations about the Stanford walking experiment; see also Marily Oppezzo and Daniel Schwartz, "Give Your Ideas Some Legs: The Positive Effect of Walking on Creative Thinking," *Journal of Experimental Psychology: Learning, Memory, and Cognition* 40:4 (July 2014), 1142–1152.

Selye describes carrying a notebook in his *Stress of My Life*, 172; Hamilton's pocket-book is mentioned in Graves, *Life of Sir William Rowan Hamilton*, 435; Lin-Manuel Miranda talks about his notebook in Milzoff, "Lin-Manuel Miranda on Jay Z, 'The West Wing,' and 18 More Things That Influenced 'Hamilton'"; Billy Wilder talks about his "black book" in James Linville, "Billy Wilder, The Art of Screenwriting No. 1," *Paris Review* 138 (Spring 1996); Ferran Adrià is quoted in Harriet Alexander, "The World of Chef Ferran Adrià," *Telegraph* (26 April 2014), http://www.telegraph.co.uk/luxury/drinking_and_dining/31813/the-world-of-chef-ferran-adrià.html; Thomas Hobbes's note-taking is described in John Aubrey, *A Brief Life of Thomas Hobbes, 1588–1679*, published in John Aubrey, *Brief Lives* (New York: Penguin Classics, 2000), ed. John Buchanan-Brown. David Hilbert's blackboard is described in Fitzgerald and James, *Mind of the Mathematician*, 46.

McClintock is quoted in Evelyn Fox Keller, *A Feeling for the Organism* (New York: Freeman, 1983), 118.

NAP

Roy Jenkins, *Churchill* (London: Macmillan, 2001), is my personal favorite one-volume biography of Winston Churchill among the vast literature on him. The War Rooms is the subject of Richard Holmes, *Churchill's Bunker: The Secret Headquarters at the Heart of Britain's Victory* (London: Profile Books, 2009). Frank Sawyers is quoted in Michael Paterson, *Winston Churchill: Personal Accounts of the Great Leader at War* (Newton Abbot, UK: David & Charles, 2005), 28. MacArthur's napping habit is described in Hiroshi Masuda and Reiko Yamamoto, *MacArthur in Asia: The General and His Staff in the Philippines, Japan, and Korea* (Ithaca, NY: Cornell University Press, 2012), quote on 282; Marshall's advice to Eisenhower is recounted in Harry Butcher, *My Three Years with Eisenhower: The Personal Diary of Captain Harry Butcher, Naval Aide to General Eisenhower, 1942–1945* (New York: Simon and Schuster, 1946).

Arthur M. Schlesinger Jr., *A Thousand Days: John F. Kennedy in the White House* (Boston: Houghton Mifflin, 1965), describes John F. Kennedy's naps. Lyndon Johnson's naps are recounted in Robert Dallek, *Flawed Giant: Lyndon Johnson and His Times, 1961–1973* (Oxford, UK: Oxford University Press, 1998).

Dayong Zhao et al., "Effects of Physical Positions on Sleep Architectures and Post-Nap Functions Among Habitual Nappers," *Biological Psychology* 83 (2010), 207–213, compares upright and horizontal napping.

Sam Weller, *The Bradbury Chronicles: The Life of Ray Bradbury* (Harper Collins, 2005), 157, describes Ray Bradbury's naps; Jonathan Franzen recounts his naps in Stephen J. Burn, "Jonathan Franzen, The Art of Fiction No. 207," *Paris Review* 195 (Winter 2010); Haruki Murakami's are in *What I Talk About When I Talk About Running*, 49–50; William Gibson's are in David Wallace-Wells, "William Gibson, The Art of Fiction No. 211," *Paris Review* 197 (Summer 2011); Mann's are in Morton, "A Talk with Thomas Mann at 80"; Stephen King's are in *On Writing*, quote on 152.

Oscar Niemeyer, *The Curves of Time: The Memoirs of Oscar Niemeyer* (London: Phaidon, 2000), is of interest on Niemeyer's schedule, as well as Philip Jodidio, *Niemeyer* (Cologne, Germany: Taschen, 2012); on Frank Lloyd Wright and Louis Kahn, see Currey, *Daily Rituals*, 131–132; Alfred Tate's quotes are from "Thomas Edison," *The Weekly Kansas City Star*, 10 August 1938, and William Dement, *The Promise of Sleep* (New York: Dell, 1999), 328; Sawyers is quoted in Paterson, *Winston Churchill*, 28. Frank Lloyd Wright's advice was reported by Maria Durrell Stone in Tafel, ed., *Frank Lloyd Wright*, 57.

On the benefits of naps in general, see Catherine Miller and Kimberly Cote, "Benefits of Napping in Healthy Adults: Impact of Nap Length, Time of Day, Age, and Experience with Napping," *Journal of Sleep Research* 18 (2009), 272–281.

See Sara Mednick, Ken Nakayama, and Robert Stickgold, "Sleep-Dependent Learning: A Nap Is as Good as a Night," *Nature Neuroscience* 6:7 (July 2003), 697–698, on naps and memory; see also Olaf Lahl et al., "An Ultra Short Episode of Sleep Is Sufficient to Promote Declarative Memory Performance," *Journal of Sleep Research* 17:1 (March 2008), 3–10; Sara C. Mednick and Sean P. A. Drummond, "Sleep: A Prescription for Insight?," *Insom* 3 (Summer 2004), 26–29. Research on rats, spatial memory and naps is in H. Freyja Ólafsdóttir et al., "Hippocampal Place Cells Construct Reward-Related Sequences Through Unexplored Space," *eLife* 4 (2015) e06063, doi: 10.7554/eLife.06063; H. Freyja Ólafsdóttir and Caswell Barry, "Spatial Cognition: Grid Cell Firing Depends on Self-Motion Cues," *Current Biology* 25:19 (2015), R827–R829; H. Freyja Ólafsdóttir, Francis Carpenter, and Caswell Barry, "Coordinated Grid and Place Cell Replay During Rest," *Nature Neuroscience* (April 2016), 1–6.

See Jennifer R. Goldschmied et al., "Napping to Modulate Frustration and Impulsivity: A Pilot Study," *Personality and Individual Differences* 86 (November 2015), 164–167, on napping and impulsivity; see also

Kathleen Vohs et al., "Ego Depletion Is Not Just Fatigue: Evidence from a Total Sleep Deprivation Experiment," *Social Psychological and Personality Science* 2:2 (March 2011), 166–173. Christopher Barnes has published several studies on sleep deprivation and its impact on decision-making: see Barnes et al., "Lack of Sleep and Unethical Behavior," *Organizational Behavior and Human Decision Processes* 115:2 (July 2011), 169–180; Brian Guina, Barnes, and Sunita Sah, "The Morality of Larks and Owls: Unethical Behavior Depends on Chronotype as Well as Time-of-Day," *Psychological Science* 25:12 (October 2014), 2272–2274; Barnes et al., "You Wouldn't Like Me When I'm Sleepy: Leader Sleep, Daily Abusive Supervision, and Work Unit Engagement," *Academy of Management Journal* 58:5 (October 2015), 1419–1437.

Mednick's work on timing naps is summarized in Sara Mednick with Mark Ehrman, *Take a Nap! Change Your Life* (New York: Workman Publishing, 2006).

Edgar Allan Poe, "Marginalia 150," *Graham's Magazine*, 28: 2 (March 1846), 116–118, describes ideas that "arise" on the "brink of sleep" on 116; Breton's description of hypnagogia is from André Breton, "What Is Surrealism?," in Herschel Browning Chipp, Peter Howard Selz, and Joshua Charles Taylor, eds., *Theories of Modern Art: A Source Book by Artists and Critics* (Berkeley, CA: University of California Press, 1968), 410; William Gibson is quoted in David Wallace-Wells, "William Gibson, The Art of Fiction No. 211"; Salvador Dalí, *Fifty Secrets of Magic Craftsmanship* (1948; repr. New York: Dover, 1992), 33–38; Bernard Ewell, "Provenance Is Everything, undated essay, Park West Gallery Dali Collection, online at http://dali.parkwestgallery.com/provenance.htm.

Michelle Carr discusses hypnagogia in her essay "How to Dream Like Salvador Dali," *Psychology Today* (20 February 2015), online at https://www.psychologytoday.com/blog/dream-factory/201502/how-dream-salvador-dali. See also E. B. Gurstelle and J. L. de Oliveira, "Daytime Parahypnagogia: A State of Consciousness That Occurs When We Almost Fall Asleep," *Medical Hypotheses* 62:2 (February 2004), 166–168; Neel V. Patel, "Sleeping On, and Dreaming Up, a Solution," *Science Online* (27 June 2014), online at http://scienceline.org/2014/06/sleeping-on-and-dreaming-up-a-solution/; Michelle Carr and Tore Nielsen, "Daydreams and Nap Dreams: Content Comparisons," *Consciousness and Cognition* 36 (2015), 196–205. For an older but still useful review of hypnagogia, see Daniel L. Schacter, "The Hypnagogic State: A Critical Review of the Literature," *Psychological Bulletin* 83:3 (1976), 452–481. Nielsen's procedure is described in Tore A. Nielsen, "A Self-Observational Study of

Spontaneous Hypnagogic Imagery Using the Upright Napping Procedure," *Imagination, Cognition and Personality* 11:4 (June 1992), 353–366.

Stop

Semi Chellas, "Matthew Weiner, The Art of Screenwriting No. 4," *Paris Review* 208 (Spring 2014), describes Allan Burns's and Matthew Weiner's practice; Roald Dahl's quote is from Dahl, *George's Marvelous Medicine* (New York: A. A. Knopf, 2002), 97; Salman Rushdie discusses his rhythm and stops in Jack Livings, "Salman Rushdie, The Art of Fiction No. 186," *Paris Review* 174 (Summer 2005); Llosa is quoted in Hunnewell and Setti, "Mario Vargas Llosa, The Art of Fiction No. 120"; Littlewood is quoted from his "The Mathematician's Art of Work," 117; Neal Stephenson discusses stopping in Laura Miller, "The Salon Interview: Neal Stephenson," *Salon* (21 April 2004), http://www.salon.com/2004/04/21/stephenson_4/; John McPhee explains why he stops in Peter Hessler, "John McPhee: The Art of Nonfiction No. 3," *Paris Review* 192 (Spring 2010); Murakami's quotes are from *What I Talk About When I Talk About Running*, 4–5.

Plimpton, "Ernest Hemingway, The Art of Fiction No. 21," has Hemingway's discussion of the subconscious; le Carré talks about sleeping on ideas in Plimpton, "John le Carré, The Art of Fiction No. 149"; Poincaré talks about unconscious work in *Foundations of Science*, 389.

Sophie Ellwood et al. "The Incubation Effect: Hatching a Solution?" *Creativity Research Journal* 21:1 (2009), 6–14, quote on 6, is of interest for the University of Sydney research, as is Jason Gallate et al., "Creative People Use Nonconscious Processes to Their Advantage," *Creativity Research Journal* 24:3 (2012), 146–151, quote on 149.

Ed Smith's observation on stopping is from Smith, "What Some People Call Idleness Is Often the Best Investment," *New Statesman* (19 July 2012), online at http://www.newstatesman.com/business/business/2012/07/what-some-people-call-idleness-often-best-investment.

Sleep

There is a large and interesting literature on sleep and its place in contemporary society—or, more often, the place that is being denied to sleep. Among recent books, Arianna Huffington's *The Sleep Revolution: Transforming Your Life, One Night at a Time* (New York: Harmony Books, 2016) is notable for its scope and informality. Jonathan Crary, *24/7: Late*

Capitalism and the Ends of Sleep (London: Verso, 2013) is more political; A. Roger Ekirch, *At Day's Close: Night in Times Past* (New York: W. W. Norton, 2005), is a fascinating historical study.

See Brooke Borel, "Do Plants Sleep?," *Popular Science* (10 March 2014), online at http://www.popsci.com/blog-network/our-modern-plagues/do -plants-sleep?, on nonhuman sleep, as well as: Jo Marchant, "Why Brainy Animals Need More REM sleep After All," *New Scientist* (19 June 2008), online at https://www.newscientist.com/article/dn14164-why-brainy -animals-need-more-rem-sleep-after-all; Andrew J. K. Phillips et al., "Mammalian Sleep Dynamics: How Diverse Features Arise from a Common Physiological Framework," *PLOS Computational Biology* (24 June 2010), doi: 10.1371/journal.pcbi.1000826.

William Dement, *The Promise of Sleep*, is the main source this account of sleep draws on. Sleep deprivation's impact on memory is described in Jutta Backhaus et al., "Impaired Declarative Memory Consolidation During Sleep in Patients with Primary Insomnia: Influence of Sleep Architecture and Nocturnal Cortisol Release," *Biological Psychiatry* 60:12 (December 2006), 1324–1330.

Lulu Xie, Maiken Nedergaard, et al., "Sleep Drives Metabolite Clearance from the Adult Brain," *Science* 342 (18 October 2013), 373–377, presents research on glial cells and the sleeping brain.

See Nita Lewis Miller, Lawrence Shattuck, and Panagiotis Matsangas, "Sleep and Fatigue Issues in Continuous Operations: A Survey of US Army Officers," *Behavioral Sleep Medicine* 9 (2011), 53–65, on sleep deprivation and the military; see also Nita Lewis Miller, Panagiotis Matsangas, and Lawrence Shattuck, "Fatigue and Its Effect on Performance in Military Environments," in James L. Szalma and Peter A. Hancock, eds., *Performance Under Stress* (Aldershot, UK: Ashgate, 2008), 231–249; Gareth Evans, "Fighting Fatigue: Cognitive Science Is Transforming Soldier Attention Spans," *Army Technology* (14 August 2013), online at http://www.army-technology.com/features /feature-fighting-fatigue-cognitive-science-soldier-attention-spans/.

See David Kenagy et al., "Dextroamphetamine Use During B-2 Combat Missions," *Aviation, Space, and Environmental Medicine* 75:5 (May 2004), 381–386, on B-2 flight crews. Mary Melfi's research is presented in James C. Miller and Mary L. Melfi, *Causes and Effects of Fatigue in Experienced Military Aircrew* (Air Force Research Laboratory, 2006), online at http://www.dtic.mil/dtic/tr/fulltext/u2/a462989.pdf. On pilots and sleep deprivation, see John A. Caldwell et al., "Fatigue Counter-measures in Aviation," *Aviation, Space and Environmental Medicine* 80:1

(January 2009), 29–59; Beth M. Hartzler, "Fatigue on the Flight Deck: The Consequences of Sleep Loss and the Benefits of Napping," *Accident Analysis and Prevention* 62 (2014), 309–318; Sigurdur Hrafn Gislason, "The Effects of ACMI Flight Crew's Long Term Outstation Hotel Stay on Accumulated Fatigue," *Transport and Aerospace Engineering* (2015), 36–41.

See Ilda Amirian, "The Impact of Sleep Deprivation on Surgeons' Performance During Night Shifts," *Danish Medical Journal* 61:9 (2014), 1–14; Syed N. Zafar et al., "The Sleepy Surgeon: Does Night-Time Surgery for Trauma Affect Mortality Outcomes?" *American Journal of Surgery* 209:4 (April 2015), 633–639; Philippa Gander et al., "Sleep Loss and Performance of Anaesthesia Trainees and Specialists," *Chronobiology International* 25:6 (2008), 1077–1091; Ilda Amirian et al., "Laparoscopic Skills and Cognitive Function Are Not Affected in Surgeons During a Night Shift," *Journal of Surgical Education* 71:4 (July–August 2014), 543–550; Mohamed Zaki Ramadan and Khalid Saad Al-Saleh, "The Association of Sleep Deprivation on the Occurrence of Errors by Nurses Who Work the Night Shift," *Current Health Sciences Journal* 40:2 (April–June 2014): 97–103; Y. S. Chang et al., "Did a Brief Nap Break Have Positive Benefits on Information Processing Among Nurses Working on the First 8-H Night Shift?," *Applied Ergonomics* 48 (May 2015), 104–108; Arlene L. Johnson et al., "Sleep Deprivation and Psychomotor Performance Among Night-Shift Nurses," *American Association of Occupational Health Nurses Journal* 58:4 (2010), 147–156 on the impact of sleep deprivation on doctors and nurses.

J. M. Harrington, "Health Effects of Shift Work and Extended Hours of Work," *Occupational and Environmental Medicine* 58:1 (2001), 68–72, describes the health effects of sleep deprivation and shift work; see also Xiaoti Lin et al., "Night-Shift Work Increases Morbidity of Breast Cancer and All-Cause Mortality: A Meta-Analysis of 16 Prospective Cohort Studies," *Sleep Medicine* 16:11 (November 2015), 1381–1387; David A. Kalmbach et al., "Shift Work Disorder, Depression, and Anxiety in the Transition to Rotating Shifts: The Role of Sleep Reactivity," *Sleep Medicine* 16:12 (December 2015), 1532–1538; Karin I. Proper et al., "The Relationship Between Shift Work and Metabolic Risk Factors: A Systematic Review of Longitudinal Studies," *American Journal of Preventive Medicine* 50:5 (May 2016) e147–e157; Chiara Dall'Ora et al., "Characteristics of Shift Work and Their Impact on Employee Performance and Wellbeing: A Literature Review," *International Journal of Nursing Studies* 57 (May 2016), 12–27.

Adam P. Spira, "Impact of Sleep on the Risk of Cognitive Decline and Dementia," *Current Opinion in Psychiatry* 27:6 (November 2014), 478–483, discusses the links between sleep deprivation and dementias; see also: Jiu-Chiuan Chen et al., "Sleep Duration, Cognitive Decline, and Dementia Risk in Older Women," *Alzheimer's and Dementia* 12:1 (January 2016), 21–33; Roberta Biundo et al., "MMSE and MoCA in Parkinson's Disease and Dementia with Lewy Bodies: A Multicenter 1-Year Follow-Up Study," *Journal of Neural Transmission* 123:4 (April 2016), 431–438.

Flaviany Ribeiro Silva et al., "Sleep on the Job Partially Compensates for Sleep Loss in Night Shift Nurses," *Chronobiology International* 23:6 (2006), 1389–1399, describes the Brazilian night nurse study.

See John A. Caldwell, J. Lynn Caldwell, and Regina M. Schmidt, "Alertness Management Strategies for Operational Contexts," *Sleep Medicine Reviews* 12 (2008), 257–273, doi: 10.1016/j.smrv.2008.01.002, for recommendations on strategic or prophylactic napping in the US military; see also Nila Joan Blackwell et al., *Leader's Guide to Soldier and Crew Endurance* (Fort Rucker, Alabama: US Army Combat Readiness Center, 2015), Hartzler, "Fatigue on the Flight Deck."

Mark Rosekind et al., "Alertness Management: Strategic Naps in Operational Settings," *Journal of Sleep Research* 4:2 (1995), 62–66, describes the 747 crew study.

See Avi Karni et al., "Dependence on REM Sleep of Overnight Improvement of a Perceptual Skill," *Science* 265 (29 July 1994), 679–682, on REM sleep and visual discrimination; more recently, see Erin J. Wamsley and Robert Stickgold, "Memory, Sleep and Dreaming: Experiencing Consolidation," *Sleep Medicine Clinic* 6:1 (March 2011), 97–108.

See Matthew P. Walker, "The Role of Slow Wave Sleep in Memory Processing," *Journal of Clinical Sleep Medicine* 5:2 supplement (April 2009), S20–S26, on slow-wave sleep and memory. On insomnia and memory, see Jutta Backhaus et al., "Impaired Declarative Memory Consolidation During Sleep in Patients with Primary Insomnia: Influence of Sleep Architecture and Nocturnal Cortisol Release," *Biological Psychiatry* 60:12 (December 2006), 1324–1330.

See Kieran C. R. Fox et al., "Dreaming as Mind Wandering: Evidence from Functional Neuroimaging and First-Person Content Reports," *Frontiers in Human Neuroscience* 4:412 (July 2013), 1–16, quote on 1, on dreams and mind-wandering.

See Sabine Lee and Gerry E. Brown, "Hans Albrecht Bethe, 2 July 1906–6 March 2005," *Biographical Memoirs of Fellows of the Royal Society*

53 (2007), 1–20, on Bethe's dreams; Linus Pauling, "The Genesis of Ideas," typed ms. dated 1961, online at http://scarc.library.oregonstate .edu/coll/pauling/calendar/1961/06/7.html#1961s2.7.tei.xml; Seaborg, quoted in "Academy of Achievement, Interview with Glenn Seaborg, September 21, 1990," http://www.achievement.org/autodoc/printmember /sea0int-1.

Simon Jenkins, "Digging It Out of the Dirt: Ben Hogan, Deliberate Practice and the Secret," *Annual Review of Golf Coaching* (2010), 7, describes golf and dreaming; on Nicklaus, see Richard Coop, *Mind Over Golf: Play Your Best By Thinking Smart* (New York: Macmillan, 1993). On sleep and dreams in creative lives, see Deirdre Barrett, *The Committee of Sleep* (New York: Crown Books, 2001).

Joseph Jastrow, *The Subconscious* (Boston: Houghton, Mifflin and Co., 1906), 94, is the source of the closing quotation; Samson and Nunn's theory is presented in David R. Samson and Charles L. Nunn, "Sleep Intensity and the Evolution of Human Cognition," *Evolutionary Anthropology: Issues, News, and Reviews* 24:6 (November/December 2015), 225–237.

RECOVERY

Harry Butcher's memoir, *My Three Years with Eisenhower: The Personal Diary of Captain Harry Butcher, Naval Aide to General Eisenhower, 1942–1945* (New York: Simon and Schuster, 1946), is the main source for the story of Eisenhower and Telegraph Hill; quotes are from 44, 76. Summersby is quoted in John Wukovits and Wesley K. Clark, *Eisenhower* (Gordonsville, VA: Palgrave Macmillan), 79.

See Zachary Ross, *Women on the Verge: The Culture of Neurasthenia in Nineteenth-Century American* (Stanford, CA: Iris & B. Gerald Cantor Center for Visual Arts, 2004), and especially David G. Schuster, *Neurasthenic Nation: America's Search for Health, Happiness, and Comfort, 1869–1920* (New Brunswick: Rutgers University Press, 2011), on neurasthenia in America. Nancy Cervetti, *S. Weir Mitchell, 1829–1914: Philadelphia's Literary Physician* (University Park: Pennsylvania State University Press, 2012) is a biography of one of the leading figures in the diagnosis of neurasthenia.

Kelly Phillips Erb, "The Real Cost of Summer Vacation: Don't Get Buried in Taxes," *Forbes* (7 July 2014), online at http://www.forbes.com /sites/kellyphillipserb/2014/07/07/the-real-cost-of-summer-vacation -dont-get-buried-in-taxes/, is the source of statistics on American vacation spending and quotes the American Express Spending & Saving Tracker:

2013 Summer Vacations (28 May 2013), online at http://about.american
express.com/news/sst/report/2013–05_Spend-and-Save-Tracker
.pdf, and BMO Private Bank's survey of millionaires and their leisure,
"BMO Private Bank Study: Affluent Americans Plan to Spend an Average of $13,000 on Vacations This Year" (press release, 21 July 2015),
https://newsroom.bmo.com/press-releases/bmo-private-bank-study
-affluent-americans-plan-to-nyse-bmo-201507211017916001. Statistics
on vacation-day use and costs of unused vacation is from Rachel Emma
Silverman, "The Price of Unused Vacation Time: $224 Billion," *Wall
Street Journal* (4 March 2015), http://blogs.wsj.com/atwork/2015/03/04
/the-cost-of-unused-vacation-time-224-billion/.

Elaine D. Eaker, Joan Pinsky, and William P. Castelli, "Myocardial
Infarction and Coronary Death Among Women: Psychosocial Predic-
tors from a 20-Year Follow-Up of Women in the Framingham Study,"
American Journal of Epidemiology 135:8 (1992), 854–864, is one study on
vacation and health; others include: Brooks Gump and Karen Matthews,
"Are Vacations Good for Your Health? The 9-Year Mortality Experience
After the Multiple Risk Factor Intervention Trial," *Psychosomatic Med-
icine* 62:5 (September–October 2000), 608–612; Chun-Chu Chen and
James F. Petrick, "Health and Wellness Benefits of Travel Experiences:
A Literature Review," *Journal of Travel Research* 52:6 (November 2013),
709–719.

Rachel Emma Silverman, "The Price of Unused Vacation Time:
$224 Billion," *Wall Street Journal* (4 March 2015), http://blogs.wsj
.com/atwork/2015/03/04/the-cost-of-unused-vacation-time-224
-billion/, estimates the cost of unused vacation time.

Cristina Queirós, Mariana Kaiseler, and António Leitão da Silva,
"Burnout as Predictor of Aggressivity Among Police Officers," *European
Journal of Policing Studies* 1:2 (December 2013), 110–135, which includes
a review of recent literature, is one of the articles on burnout mentioned
here; others include: Tait D. Shanafelt et al., "Burnout and Career Satisfaction Among American Surgeons," *Annals of Surgery* 250:3 (September 2009), 463–471; Tait D. Shanafelt and C. M. Balch, "Combating
Stress and Burnout in Surgical Practice: A Review," *Advances in Surgery*
44 (2010), 29–47; Tait D. Shanafelt et al., "Burnout and Medical Errors Among American Surgeons," *Annals of Surgery* 251:6 (June 2010),
995–1000; Tait D. Shanafelt et al., "Avoiding Burnout: The Personal
Health Habits and Wellness Practices of US Surgeons," *Annals of Surgery* 255:4 (April 2012), 625–633; Tait D. Shanafelt et al., "Burnout and
Satisfaction with Work-Life Balance Among US Physicians Relative to

the General US Population," *Archives of Internal Medicine* 172:18 (2012), 1377–1385. The Methodist clergy study is the *2014 Statewide Survey of United Methodist Clergy in North Carolina* (Duke Clergy Health Initiative, 2014).

Wayne Oates coined the term *workaholic* in *Confessions of a Workaholic: The Facts About Work Addiction* (New York: World Publishing Company, 1971); Oates describes his discovery of burnout in his autobiography, *The Struggle to Be Free: My Story and Your Story* (Philadelphia: Westminster Press, 1983).

On vacations and inspiration, see Anna Almendrala, "Lin-Manuel Miranda: It's 'No Accident' Hamilton Came to Me on Vacation," *Huffington Post* (23 June 2016), online at http://www.huffingtonpost.com/entry /lin-manuel-miranda-says-its-no-accident-hamilton-inspiration-struck -on-vacation_us_576c136ee4b0b489bb0ca7c2?; Lyman Spitzer, "Dreams, Stars, and Electrons," *Annual Review of Astronomy and Astrophysics* 27 (1989), 1–17; on Systrom and the start-up survey, see Hollie Slade, "Want a Brilliant Idea for a Startup? Go on Vacation," *Forbes* (30 June 2014), online at http://www.forbes.com/sites/hollieslade/2014/06/30/want-a-brilliant -idea-for-a-startup-go-on-vacation/; on Rafa Soto and OmmWriter, see Pang, *The Distraction Addiction*, 70.

Sabine Sonnentag has published dozens of articles with a number of colleagues; a good introduction to her work, and to the concepts of detachment and recovery, are Sabine Sonnentag, "Recovery, Work Engagement, and Proactive Behavior: A New Look at the Interface Between Nonwork and Work," *Journal of Applied Psychology* 88:3 (2003), 518–528, and Charlotte Fritz and Sonnentag, "Recovery, Health, and Job Performance: Effects of Weekend Experiences," *Journal of Occupational Health Psychology* 10:3 (2005), 187–199. On programmers, see Maike E. Debus, Werner Deutsch, Sabine Sonnentag, Fridtjof W. Nussbeck, "Making Flow Happen: The Effects of Being Recovered on Work-Related Flow Between and Within Days," *Journal of Applied Psychology* 99:3 (2014); Sabine Sonnentag and Charlotte Fritz, "The Recovery Experience Questionnaire: Development and Validation of a Measure for Assessing Recuperation and Unwinding from Work," *Journal of Occupational Health Psychology* 12:3 (2007), 204–221, quote on 206; on physicians and nurses, see Sabine Sonnentag and Fred R. H. Zijlstra, "Job Characteristics and Off-Job Activities as Predictors of Need for Recovery, Well-Being, and Fatigue," *Journal of Applied Psychology* 91:2 (2006), 330–350. An interesting comparative study of evening-hours use among business professionals is being undertaken by Jeremy Schulz and is described in two articles:

"Talk of Work: Transatlantic Divergences in Justifications for Hard Work Among French, Norwegian, and American Professionals," *Theory and Society* 41:6 (November 2012), 603–634, and "Winding Down the Workday: Zoning the Evening Hours in Paris, Oslo, and San Francisco," *Qualitative Sociology* 38:3 (September 2015), 235–259.

Mihaly Csikszentmihalyi's major work on flow is *Flow: The Psychology of Optimal Experience*, rev. ed. (London: Rider, 2002).

See Jack Copeland, *Colossus: The Secrets of Bletchley Park's Code-Breaking Computers* (Oxford, UK: Oxford University Press, 2006), on chess players and Bletchley Park.

See Dalia Etzion, Dov Eden, and Yael Lapidot, "Relief from Job Stressors and Burnout: Reserve Service as a Respite," *Journal of Applied Psychology* 83:4 (August 1998), 577–585 on detachment, recovery, and military experience; see also Trevor T. Sthultz, "Military Deployments as a Respite from Burnout: An Analysis of Gender and Family" (M.S. thesis, Air Force Institute of Technology, 2004); S. Ryan Johnson, "Effects of Deployments on Homestation Job Stress and Burnout" (M.S. thesis, Air Force Institute of Technology, 2005); Patrick A. Horsman, "Is a Change as Good as a Rest?: Investigating Part-Time Reserve Service as a Method of Stress Recovery" (M.A. thesis in Applied Psychology, Saint Mary's University, 2011).

See Mina Westman and Dalia Etzion, "The Impact of Short Overseas Business Trips on Job Stress and Burnout," *Applied Psychology* 51:4 (October 2002), 582–592, on work-related travel and recovery; see also: Mina Westman, Dalia Etzion, and Shoshi Chen, "Are Business Trips a Unique Kind of Respite?" in Sabine Sonnentag, Daniel Ganster, and Pamela L. Perrewé, eds., *Current Perspectives on Job-Stress Recovery*, Research in Occupational Stress and Well-Being, volume 7 (Bingley, UK: JAI Press/Elsevier Science, 2009), 167–204; Sabine Sonnentag and Eva Natter, "Flight Attendants' Daily Recovery from Work: Is There No Place Like Home?" *International Journal of Stress Management* 11:4 (2004), 366–391; Ben J. Searle, "Detachment from Work in Airport Hotels: Issues for Pilot Recovery," *Aviation Psychology and Applied Human Factors* 2:1 (2012), 20–24.

Ben Kazez described his musical and programming interests in an interview with author, 1 June 2015. On smartphones and detachment, see Young Ah Park, Charlotte Fritz, and Steve M. Jex, "Relationships Between Work-Home Segmentation and Psychological Detachment from Work: The Role of Communication Technology Use at Home," *Journal of Occupational Health Psychology* 16:4 (2011), 457–467;

Katherine Richardson and Cynthia Thompson, "High Tech Tethers and Work-Family Conflict: A Conservation of Resources Approach," *Engineering Management Research* 1:1 (2012), 29–43; Sophie Ward and Gail Steptoe-Warren, "A Conservation of Resources Approach to Blackberry Use, Work-Family Conflict and Well-Being: Job Control and Psychological Detachment from Work as Potential Mediators," *Engineering Management Research* 3:1 (2014), 8–23; Jan Dettmers et al., "Extended Work Availability and Its Relation with Start-of-Day Mood and Cortisol," *Journal of Occupational Health Psychology* 21:1 (January 2016), 105–118.

See Mina Westman and Dov Eden, "Effects of a Respite from Work on Burnout: Vacation Relief and Fade-Out," *Journal of Applied Psychology* 82:4 (August 1997), 516–527, on the duration of vacation and respite benefits; see also Mina Westman and Dalia Etzion, "The Impact of Vacation and Job Stress on Burnout and Absenteeism," *Psychology & Health* 16:5 (2001), 595–606; Jessica de Bloom et al., "Effects of Vacation from Work on Health and Well-Being: Lots of Fun, Quickly Gone," *Work & Stress* 24:2 (April 2010), 196–216; Jessica de Bloom, Sabine Geurts, and Michiel Kompier, "Vacation from Work as Prototypical Recovery Opportunity," *Gedrag & Organisatie* 23:4 (December 2010), 333–349; Jana Kühnel and Sabine Sonnentag, "How Long Do You Benefit from Vacation?: A Closer Look at the Fade-Out of Vacation Effects," *Journal of Organizational Behavior* 32:1 (January 2011), 125–143; Jeroen Nawijn, "Happiness Through Vacationing: Just a Temporary Boost or Long-Term Benefits?" *Journal of Happiness Studies* 12:4 (August 2011), 651–665; Mina Westman and Dalia Etzion, "The Impact of Vacation and Job Stress on Burnout and Absenteeism," *Psychology & Health* 16:5 (2001), 595–606; Dalia Etzion, "Annual Vacation: Duration of Relief from Job Stressors," *Anxiety, Stress, and Coping* 16:2 (June 2003), 213–226. De Bloom is quoted in Sumatra Reddy, "The Smartest Way to Take a Vacation: Scientists Study How to Get the Most Benefits in Health and Well-Being from a Getaway," *Wall Street Journal* (20 July 2015), online at http://www.wsj.com/articles/smartest-way-to-take-a-vacation-1437406680.

Butcher's quotes are from *My Three Years with Eisenhower*, 88, 116.

Exercise

Robert S. Root-Bernstein, Maurine Bernstein, and Helen Garnier, "Correlations Between Avocations, Scientific Style, Work Habits, and Professional Impact of Scientists," *Creativity Research Journal* 8:2 (1995) 115–137, quotes from 125, is the Eiduson study follow-up.

Pat Haden is a well-known Rhodes Scholar and football player, but the others mentioned in the text are less famous: see Dennis J. Hutchinson, *The Man Who Once Was Whizzer White: A Portrait of Justice Byron R. White* (New York: Free Press, 1998); Aaron Gordon, "The Rejection of Myron Rolle," *SB Nation* (12 February 2014), http://www.sbnation.com/longform/2014/2/12/5401774/myron-rolle-profile-florida-state-football-nfl-rhodes-scholar; Frank Ryan's career as an athlete and mathematician is described in Jonas Fortune, "A Man of Two Worlds," *Case Western Reserve Magazine* (Fall 2012), online at http://newartsci.case.edu/magazine/fall-2012/a-man-of-two-worlds/; Urschel talks about his dual life in Stephen D. Miller, "'I Plan to Be a Great Mathematician': An NFL Offensive Lineman Shows He's One of Us," *Notices of the AMS* 63:2 (February 2016), 148–151.

On noted scientist-athletes, see J. J. O'Connor and E. F. Robertson, "Harald August Bohr," *MacTutor History of Mathematics Archive*, online at http://www-history.mcs.st-andrews.ac.uk/Biographies/Bohr_Harald.html; Susan Quinn, *Marie Curie: A Life* (New York: Simon & Schuster, 1995); Kathleen Rowe, "MIT Hurdler was Victor/Chronicler of 1896 Olympics," *MIT News* (July 18, 1996), http://news.mit.edu/1996/olymp1896-curtis (on Thomas Pelham Curtis); Roger Bannister, *Twin Tracks: The Autobiography* (London: Robson Press, 2015); Lillian Hoddeson, *True Genius: The Life and Science of John Bardeen: The Only Winner of Two Nobel Prizes in Physics* (Washington, DC: Joseph Henry Press, 2002); George G. Brownlee, *Fred Sanger, Double Nobel Laureate: A Biography* (Cambridge, UK: Cambridge University Press, 2014); Louise Rafkin, "Sitting on Top of the World," *San Francisco Chronicle* (30 December 2001), http://www.sfgate.com/bayarea/article/SITTING-ON-TOP-OF-THE-WORLD-Sarah-Gerhardt-on-3307271.php (on Sarah Gerhardt).

Andrew Warwick's terrific book *Masters of Theory: Cambridge and the Rise of Mathematical Physics* (Chicago: University of Chicago Press, 2003) is the source of my account of the Cambridge wranglers; quotes are from Warwick, "Exercising the Student Body: Mathematics and Athletics in Victorian Cambridge," in Christopher Lawrence and Steven Shapin, eds., *Science Incarnate: Historical Embodiments of Natural Knowledge* (Chicago: University of Chicago Press, 1998), 288–323, on 294, 309, 314. The wranglers' athleticism was partly a defense against the mental strain of studying mathematics: see Alice Jenkins, "Mathematics and Mental Health in Early Nineteenth-Century England," *BSHM Bulletin: Journal of the British Society for the History of Mathematics* 25:2 (2010), 92–103.

Peter Harman and Simon Mitton, eds., *Cambridge Scientific Minds* (Cambridge, UK: Cambridge University Press, 2002) provides an overview of science at Cambridge through the biographies of its leading figures.

John Carew Eccles, *Sherrington, His Life and Thought* (Berlin: Springer-Verlag, 1979), is of interest on Sherrington and his circle; quote is from "Sir Charles Sherrington—Biographical," *Nobel Lectures, Physiology or Medicine 1922–1941* (Amsterdam: Elsevier, 1965), online at http://www.nobelprize.org/nobel_prizes/medicine/laureates/1932/sherrington-bio.html; see also Wilder Penfield, *No Man Alone: A Neurosurgeon's Story* (Boston: Little, Brown & Co., 1977); Jefferson Lewis, *Something Hidden: A Biography of Wilder Penfield* (New York: Doubleday, 1981), a revealing biography by one of his grandchildren; Eric Lax, *The Mold in Dr. Florey's Coat: The Story of the Penicillin Miracle* (New York: Henry Holt and Co., 2004). On Fulton, see Jack D. Pressman, *Last Resort: Psychosurgery and the Limits of Medicine* (Cambridge, UK: Cambridge University Press, 1998), and Michael Bliss, "The Last Latchkeyer: The Tragedy of John Fulton" (paper presented at the meeting of the American Osler Society, Montreal, 1 May 2007), quote on 4 (my thanks to Dr. Bliss for sharing a copy of this piece, and for illuminating Fulton's rather Gothic story); Mary R. Mennis, *The Book of Eccles: A Portrait of Sir John Eccles, Australian Nobel Laureate and Scientist, 1903–1997* (Queensland: Lalong Enterprises, 2003).

See E. M. Tansey, "Working with C. S. Sherrington, 1918–24," *Notes and Records of the Royal Society of London* 62:1 (20 March 2008), 123–130, on Thomas Graham Brown; Brown's own laboratory manager observed that "the big trouble with him was he lost interest in physiology when he got interested in mountaineering." On scientists and mountain climbing in the nineteenth century, see Bruce Hevly, "The Heroic Science of Glacier Motion," *Osiris* 11 (1996), 66–86. On physicists and mountain climbing, see Emilio Segrè, *A Mind Always in Motion: The Autobiography of Emilio Segrè* (Berkeley, CA: University of California Press, 1993); Emilio Segrè, *Enrico Fermi, Physicist* (Chicago: University of Chicago Press, 1970); Laura Fermi, *Atoms in the Family: My Life with Enrico Fermi* (Chicago: University of Chicago Press, 1954); Peter Goodchild, *Edward Teller: The Real Dr. Strangelove* (London: Weidenfeld & Nicolson, 2004); Victor Weisskopf, *The Joy of Insight: Passions of a Physicist* (New York: Basic Books, 1991), quote on 18. On Los Alamos, the outdoors, and sports, see Mark Fiege, "The Atomic Scientists, the Sense of Wonder, and the Bomb," *Environmental History* 12:3 (2007), 578–613; Jennet Conant, *109 East Palace: Robert Oppenheimer and the Secret City of Los Alamos* (New York: Simon & Schuster, 2005); Jon Hunner, *Inventing*

Los Alamos: The Growth of an Atomic Community (Norman, OK: University of Oklahoma Press, 2004). Donald Osterbrock, "Rudolph Leo Bernhard Minkowski," *Biographical Memoirs of the National Academy of Sciences* 54 (1983), 270–299; Alfred Stöckli, *Fritz Zwicky: An Extraordinary Astrophysicist* (Cambridge, UK: Cambridge Scientific Publishers, 2011); "Steve Giddings," *Physics Central*, http://www.physicscentral.com /explore/people/giddings.cfm; George Johnson, "A Passion for Physical Realms, Minute and Massive," *New York Times* (20 February 2001), online at http://www.nytimes.com/2001/02/20/science/a-passion-for-physical -realms-minute-and-massive.html (on Lisa Randall).

My account of Franklin's climbing draws mainly on Brenda Maddox, *Rosalind Franklin: The Dark Lady of DNA* (London: Harper Collins, 2003); Jenifer Glynn, *My Sister Rosalind Franklin* (Oxford, UK: Oxford University Press, 2012); and also Anne Sayre, *Rosalind Franklin and DNA* (New York: Norton, 1975). Franklin was a lifelong athlete: she played cricket, hockey, and tennis as a student at St Paul's Girls' School and was a capable cyclist.

See Karsten Mueller et al., "Physical Exercise in Overweight to Obese Individuals Induces Metabolic- and Neurotrophic-Related Structural Brain Plasticity," *Frontiers in Human Neuroscience* 9:372 (July 2015), doi: 10.3389/fnhum.2015.00372, for scientific research exploring the influence of exercise on cognition and the brain; see also Christiane D. Wrann et al., "Exercise Induces Hippocampal BDNF Through a PGC-1α/ FNDC5 Pathway," *Cell Metabolism* 18:5 (November 2013), 649–659; Andrew S. Whiteman et al., "Interaction Between Serum BDNF and Aerobic Fitness Predicts Recognition Memory in Healthy Young Adults," *Behavioural Brain Research* 259 (2014), 302–312; Leoni Bolz, Stefanie Heigele, and Josef Bischofberger, "Running Improves Pattern Separation During Novel Object Recognition," *Brain Plasticity* 1:1 (2015), 129–145; Miriam S. Nokia et al., "Physical Exercise Increases Adult Hippocampal Neurogenesis in Male Rats Provided It Is Aerobic and Sustained," *Journal of Physiology* 594:7 (1 April 2016), 1855–1873; David M. Blanchette et al., "Aerobic Exercise and Cognitive Creativity: Immediate and Residual Effects," *Creativity Research Journal* 17:2/3 (2005), 257–264; Lorenza S. Colzato et al., "The Impact of Physical Exercise on Convergent and Divergent Thinking," *Frontiers in Human Neuroscience* 7 (December 2013), 824.

Murakami describes running "in a void" in *What I Talk About When I Talk About Running*, 16–17.

David Attwell and Simon B. Laughlin, "An Energy Budget for Signaling in the Grey Matter of the Brain," *Journal of Cerebral Blood Flow and Metabolism* 21:10 (October 2001), 1133–1145, offers the comparison of energy consumption by firing neurons and by firing leg muscles ("signaling-related energy use of 30 μmol ATP/g/min is equal to that in human leg muscle running the marathon"). On aerobic activity and its benefits, see K. Hötting et al., "Differential Cognitive Effects of Cycling Versus Stretching/Coordination Training in Middle-Aged Adults," *Health Psychology* 31 (2012), 145–55; Tina D. Hoang et al., "Effect of Early Adult Patterns of Physical Activity and Television Viewing on Midlife Cognitive Function," *JAMA Psychiatry* 73:1 (2016), 73–79; Marcus Richards, Rebecca Jane Hardy, and Michael E. J. Wadsworth, "Does Active Leisure Protect Cognition? Evidence from a National Birth Cohort," *Social Science and Medicine* 56 (2003), 785–792.

Murakami describes writing as manual labor in *What I Talk About When I Talk About Running*, 79; Shinya Yamanaka writes about marathon running in "Ekiden to iPS Cells," *Nature Medicine* 15 (2009), 1145–1148; Michaeleen Doucleff, "I'm A Runner: Wolfgang Ketterle, Ph.D.," *Runner's World* (December 2009), online at http://www.runnersworld.com/celebrity-runners/im-a-runner-wolfgang-ketterle-phd.

On chess and exercise, see Agnieszka Fornal-Urban and Anna Kęska, "Physical Fitness of Young Chess Players," *Chess Base* (23 June 2010), http://en.chessbase.com/post/physical-fitne-of-young-che-players; Tim Hanke, "Physical Fitness Promotes Mental Fitness," *Chess Improver* (30 April 2013), http://chessimprover.com/physical-fitness-promotes-mental-fitness/; Viswanathan Krishnaswamy, "Importance of Physical Fitness in Chess," *Daily Mail* (15 November 2013), online at http://www.daily mail.co.uk/indiahome/indianews/article-2508201/Carlsen-draws-blood-beating-Indian-chess-star-Anand-Chennai-fifth-game-58-moves.html; Christopher Bergland, "Checkmate!: Winning Life Strategies of a Chess Grandmaster," *Psychology Today* (7 May 2013), http://www.psychologytoday.com/blog/the-athletes-way/201305/checkmate-winning-life-strategies-chess-grandmaster; Seth Stevenson, "Grandmaster Clash," *Slate* (18 September 2014), http://www.slate.com/articles/sports/sports_nut/2014/09/sinquefield_cup_one_of_the_most_amazing_feats_in_chess_history_just_happened.single.html; Miles Hinson, "Chexercise: Chess and Physical Fitness," *Daily Princetonian* (19 October 2014), http://dailyprincetonian.com/sports/2014/10/chexercise-chess-and-physical-fitness/; Jennifer Shahade, "On Chess: Physical

Fitness Becomes Increasingly Important for Top-Level Players," *St. Louis Public Radio* (21 January 2015), http://news.stlpublicradio.org/post/chess -physical-fitness-becomes-increasingly-important-top-level-players. See Arnold Bakker et al., "Workaholism and Daily Recovery: A Day Reconstruction Study of Leisure Activities," *Journal of Organizational Behavior* 34 (2013), 87–107, on exercise, stress, and resilience; see also Tait Shanafelt et al., "Avoiding Burnout: The Personal Health Habits and Wellness Practices of US Surgeons," *Annals of Surgery* 255:4 (April 2012), 625–633; Michael G. Poulsen et al., "Recovery Experience and Burnout in Cancer Workers in Queensland," *European Journal of Oncology Nursing* 19:1 (February 2015), 23–28. Barack Obama's exercise regimen and its place in his day are described in Reggie Love, *Power Forward: My Presidential Education* (New York: Simon and Schuster, 2015); on Kagan and Ginsberg, Ann E. Marimow, "Personal Trainer Bryant Johnson's Clients Include Two Supreme Court Justices," *Washington Post* (19 March 2013), http://www.washingtonpost.com/style/personal-trainer-bryant-johnsons -clients-includetwo-supreme-court-justices/2013/03/19/ea884018– 86a1–11e2–98a3-b3db6b9ac586_story.html, and Jeffrey Rosen, "Ruth Bader Ginsburg Is an American Hero," *New Republic* (28 September 2014), http://www.newrepublic.com/article/119578 /ruth-bader-ginsburg-interview-retirement-feminists-jazzercise.

Alan Turing's athletic life is described in Andrew Hodges, *Alan Turing: The Enigma* (New York: Simon and Schuster, 1983), quote on 370.

Judith Strada, "Surf's Up! And Look Who's Hangin' 10," *San Diego Magazine* (17 September 2007), http://www.sandiegomagazine .com/San-Diego-Magazine/August-1996/Surfs-Up-And-Look -Whos-Hangin-10/, includes the quote from Donald Cram; Nelson Mandela, *Long Walk to Freedom: The Autobiography of Nelson Mandela* (Boston: Back Bay, 1995), quote on 490.

Maria A. I. Åberg et al., "Cardiovascular Fitness Is Associated with Cognition in Young Adulthood," *Proceedings of the National Academy of Sciences* 106:49 (8 December 2009) 20906–20911, is the Swedish longitudinal study; the American veterans study is Kevin M. Kniffin, Brian Wansink, and Mitsuru Shimizu, "Sports at Work: Anticipated and Persistent Correlates of Participation in High School Athletics," *Journal of Leadership & Organizational Studies* 22:2 (2015), 217–230; on women executives and sports, see Ernst & Young, "Female Executives Say Participation in Sport Helps Accelerate Leadership and Career Potential," (news release, 10 October 2014), http://www.ey.com/GL/en/Newsroom/News-releases /news-female-executives-say-participation-in-sport-helps-accelerate

—leadership-and-career-potential; Nanette Fondas, "Research: More Than Half of Top Female Execs Were College Athletes," *Harvard Business Review* (9 October 2014), https://hbr.org/2014/10/research-more -than-half-of-female-execs-were-college-athletes.

See Qi Sun et al., "Physical Activity at Midlife in Relation to Successful Survival in Women at Age 70 Years or Older," *Archives of Internal Medicine* 170:2 (2010), 194–201, on physical activity and cognitive ability in aging populations; see also Claire Joanne Steves et al., "Kicking Back Cognitive Ageing: Leg Power Predicts Cognitive Ageing After Ten Years in Older Female Twins," *Gerontology* 62:2 (2016), 138–149; Ian J. Deary et al., "The Lothian Birth Cohort 1936: A Study to Examine Influences on Cognitive Ageing from Age 11 to Age 70 and Beyond," *BMC Geriatrics* 7:28 (December 2007), 1–12; Alan J. Gow et al., "Neuroprotective Lifestyles and the Aging Brain: Activity, Atrophy, and White Matter Integrity," *Neurology* 79 (2012), 1802–1808; Mark Hamer, Kim L. Lavoie, and Simon L. Bacon, "Taking Up Physical Activity in Later Life and Healthy Ageing: The English Longitudinal Study of Ageing," *British Journal of Sports Medicine* 48 (2014), 239–243; Agnieszka Burzynska et al., "White Matter Integrity, Hippocampal Volume, and Cognitive Performance of a World-Famous Nonagenarian Track-and-Field Athlete," *Neurocase* 22:2 (March 2016), 135–144.

See Nicholas Fox Weber, *Le Corbusier* (New York: A. A. Knopf, 2008); Desmond and Moore, *Darwin*; and the materials on Sherrington and his students listed earlier on the elderly lives of physically active creatives.

Deep Play

Lindsay Lawlor quotes are all from a telephone interview with the author, 4 June 2015.

Clifford Geertz popularized the concept of deep play (among academics at least) in his now-classic "Deep Play: Notes on the Balinese Cockfight," *Daedalus* 134:4 (Fall 2005), 56–86. Cultural anthropologists will note that I'm not using the concept in precisely the same way Geertz does, but they'll be the only ones.

Norman Maclean describes playing billiards with Albert Michelson in "Billiards Is a Good Game," *University of Chicago Magazine* (Summer 1975), online at http://mag.uchicago.edu/science-medicine/billiards-good -game. Like everything Maclean wrote, it's well worth reading, as he himself noted in Nick O'Connell, "Haunted by Waters: A Talk with Norman

Maclean," *The Writer's Workshop Review* (28 March 2009), http://www.the writersworkshopreview.net/article.cgi?article_id=14. Dorothy Michelson Livingston, *The Master of Light: A Biography of Albert A. Michelson* (New York: Scribner, 1973) is an accessible biography by one of Michelson's daughters. Among the many obituaries written of Michelson, two by longtime colleagues are the best: Henry Gale, "Albert Michelson," *Astrophysical Journal* 74:1 (July 1931), 1–9, and Robert Millikan, "Albert Abraham Michelson, 1852–1931," *Biographical Memoirs of the National Academy of Sciences* 19 (1938), 119–46; Millikan quotes Michelson's wife on 128.

Churchill's *Painting as a Pastime* offers the clearest account of his artistic life; quotes are from 7, 27, 86, 61, 48, 46, 48, 53, 46. The publication of the book in the United States, according to art historian Kim Grant, helped spur an interest in amateur painting in the 1950s: see Kim Grant, "'Paint and Be Happy': The Modern Artist and the Amateur Painter—A Question of Distinction," *Journal of American Culture* 34:3 (September 2011), 289–303.

See Silvanus Phillips Thompson, *The Life of Lord Kelvin*, vol. 2 (repr. Providence, RI: AMS Chelsea Publishing, American Mathematical Society, 2005), quote on 597, on William Thomson and the *Lalla Rookh*. Industrial designer Jack Kelley described his sailing in an interview with the author, 16 March 2015. On Britton Chance's career as a sailor, see Evan Gillingham, "Sailing by Chance," *Motor Boating* (April 1967), 88–90, 92, 94; the quote from former student Les Dutton describing Britton Chance's transition from scientist to sailor is from a December 10, 2010, remembrance on http://www.brittonchance.org/?page_id=30; Chance describes the effect of the Olympics on his research in Nick Zagorski, "Britton Chance: Former Olympian and Pioneer in Enzyme Kinetics and Functional Spectroscopy," *ASBMB Today* (July 2009), 32–36, quote on 34.

Viktor Frankl discusses mountain climbing in his *Recollections: An Autobiography* (New York: Insight Books, 1997), quote on 42. Christof Koch's climbing is the subject of Karen Heyman, "Christof Koch's Ascent," *The Scientist* (14 July 2003), http://www.the-scientist.com/?articles.view/articleNo/14931/title/Christof-Koch-s-Ascent/; quotes are from Kevin Berger, "Ingenious: Christof Koch," *Nautilis* (6 November 2014), http://nautil.us/issue/19/illusions/ingenious-christof-koch. Henry Kendall describes his climbing in his Nobel Prize speech: "Henry W. Kendall—Biographical," in Tore Frängsmyr, ed., *The Nobel Prizes 1990* (Stockholm: Nobel Foundation, 1991), online at

http://www.nobelprize.org/nobel_prizes/physics/laureates/1990/kendall
-bio.html, and in an interview conducted by John Rawlings, 6 March
1997 and 13 February 1998 (Stanford Oral History Project, SC1018/1/7,
Stanford University Special Collections); Kendall's account of the world
as an "astonishingly beautiful place" is quoted in John Rawlings, *The Stanford Alpine Club* (Stanford, CA: Stanford University Libraries and CLSI
Publications, 1999), 104.

John Gill is quoted in Jon Krakauer, *Eiger Dreams: Ventures Among
Men and Mountains* (1990; repr. New York: Anchor Books, 1997), 18.
On other scientists, see J. E. Littlewood, "The Mathematician's Art of
Work," *Mathematical Intelligencer* 1:2 (June 1978), 112–119; Alan Hodg-
kin, "Edgar Douglas Adrian," *Biographical Memoirs of Fellows of the Royal
Society* 25 (1979), 1–73; Andrew Hodges, *Alan Turing: The Enigma* (New
York: Simon and Schuster, 1983); "Lyman Spitzer, 1914–1997," *Ameri-
can Alpine Club Publications* (1997), online at http://publications.american
alpineclub.org/articles/12199840900/print.

Nicole LeBrasseur, "Louis Reichardt: The Long Climb to Science's
Summits," *Journal of Cell Biology* 186:5 (September 2009), 634–635, is
one source of the Reichardt quotes; the others are: "Louis Reichardt: Expeditions in Science and Mountaineering," *iBiology* (April 2012), http://
www.ibiology.org/ibiomagazine/issue-7/louis-reichardt-expedition-in
-science-and-mountaineering.html; and Reichardt, "Lessons from K2
and Everest for Life in Science and the World," *Harvard-Radcliffe Class
of 1964 50th Reunion Brief Talks*, online at http://hr1964.org/reichardt
.htm. The description of Reichardt is from Eric Perlman, "Professor Go-
rilla," *Backpacker* (September 1986), 88.

Richard G. Mitchell, *Mountain Experience: The Psychology and Sociology of Adventure* (Chicago: University of Chicago Press, 1983) is a good
academic study of the experience of climbing and includes a discussion of
scientists' attraction to climbing. Michael Useem, Jerry Useem, and Paul
Asel, eds., *Upward Bound: Nine Original Accounts of How Business Leaders Reached Their Summits* (New York: Crown Business, 2003) and Chris
Warner and Don Schmincke, *High Altitude Leadership: What the World's
Most Forbidding Peaks Teach Us About Success* (San Francisco: Wiley,
2009) extract lessons for corporate leadership from mountain climbing.

Wilder Penfield describes his life as an author in *The Second Career*
(New York: Little, Brown & Co., 1963); Lewis, *Something Hidden*, also
is valuable.

James Herriot's life and work are the subject of Graham Lord, *James
Herriot: The Life of a Country Vet* (New York: Carroll and Graf Publishers,

1997), and Jim Wight, *The Real James Herriot: A Memoir of My Father* (New York: Ballantine, 2001). Bram Stoker and the authorship of Dracula are discussed in Barbara Belford, *Bram Stoker: A Biography of the Author of "Dracula"* (New York: Knopf, 1996), and Jim Steinmeyer, *Who was Dracula?: Bram Stoker's Trail of Blood* (New York: Jeremy Tarcher, 2013). Coincidentally, Stoker's retreat to Cruden Bay put him just a few miles from Newburgh, Scotland, where Thomas Mitchell would give the talks that became *Essays on Life*. My main source on Tolkien is Humphrey Carpenter, *J. R. R. Tolkien: A Biography* (1977; repr. Boston: Houghton Mifflin, 2000).

Maclean, "Billiards Is a Good Game," is the source of Michelson's quote in the concluding section; Root-Bernstein is from Root-Bernstein, Maurine Bernstein, and Helen Garnier, "Correlations Between Avocations, Scientific Style, Work Habits, and Professional Impact of Scientists," 132, 127.

Sabbaticals

Mar Abad, "Sagmeister: 'Variety Makes You Happier,'" *Foundation Telefonica* (2 July 2014), http://ferranadria.fundaciontelefonica.com/en /sagmeister-variety-makes-happier/, discusses Sagmeister's sabbaticals; see also Gina Trapani, "Burned Out? Take a Creative Sabbatical," *Harvard Business Review* (20 October 2009), https://hbr.org/2009/10/increase -your-productivity-by.html. The quote on misery is from Till Huber, "On Being a Designer: An Interview with Stefan Sagmeister," *Sturm und Drang* (1 May 2015), https://sturmunddrang.de/en/digest/i-was-looking -for-something-meaningful-to-design-interview-with-stefan-sagmeister/.

Harriet Alexander, "Ferran Adria Interview: The Culinary Wizard on Life After el Bulli," *The Telegraph* (29 January 2011), http://www.telegraph .co.uk/news/worldnews/europe/spain/8290685/Ferran-Adria-interview- The-culinary-wizard-on-life-after-el-Bulli.html, describes Ferran Adrià's sabbaticals; see also Ren McKnight, "Exit Interview: Ferran Adrià," *GQ* (27 July 2011), http://www.gq.com/story/ferran-adria-exit-interview -el-bulli; John Walsh, "The Last Supper: El Bulli Closes Its Doors," *The Independent* (22 October 2011), http://www.independent.co.uk/life-style /food-and-drink/features/the-last-supper-el-bulli-closes-its-doors -2327826.html; Sadie Stein, "The Remarkable Ambition and Chaos of Ferran Adrià's El Bulli Lab," *Bon Appétit* (14 May 2015), http://www .bonappetit.com/people/chefs/article/el-bulli-lab-ferran-adria.

Robert A. Guth, "In Secret Hideaway, Bill Gates Ponders Microsoft's Future," *Wall Street Journal* (28 March 2005), online at http://www .wsj.com/articles/SB111196625830690477, describes Gates's think week; see also Darryl K. Taft, "What Is Bill Gates Thinking?," *eweek* (29 March 2004), http://www.eweek.com/c/a/Windows/What-Is-Bill-Gates -Thinking. Other corporate sabbaticals are described in Michael Karnjanaprakorn, "How Skillshare's CEO Cultivates and Applies Creativity (Taking Cues from Bill Gates and Chuck Close)," *Fast Company* (26 February 2014) http://www.fastcompany.com/3024934/business-simplified /how-skillshares-ceo-cultivates-and-applies-creativity-taking-cues -from-b; Elizabeth Pagano and Barbara Pagano, "The Virtues and Challenges of a Long Break," *Journal of Accountancy* 207:2 (February 2009), 46– 51; Rosabeth Moss Kanter, "Should Leaders Go on Vacation?," *Harvard Business Review* (15 August 2011), https://hbr.org/2011/08/should-leaders -go-on-vacation.html; Tanner Christensen, "Why You Need a 'Think Week' Like Bill Gates," *99u* (10 March 2014), http://99u.com/workbook /23511/why-you-need-a-think-week-like-bill-gates; Rebecca Greenfield, "Why You Should Pay Employees to Take a Sabbatical," *Fast Company* (1 October 2014), http://www.fastcompany.com/3036344/my-creative-life/why-you-should-pay-employees-to-take-a-sabbatical; "Reflections from a CEO Sabbatical," *Polymer Solutions* (15 December 2015), https:// www.polymersolutions.com/blog/reflections-from-a-ceo-sabbatical/; Peter Strozniak, "Iowa League CEO Discusses Four-Month Sabbatical," *Credit Union Times* (9 February 2016), http://www.cutimes.com /2016/02/09/iowa-league-ceo-discusses-four-month-sabbatical.

See Deborah S. Linnell and Tim Wolfred, *Creative Disruption: Sabbaticals for Capacity Building & Leadership Development in the Nonprofit Sector* (Third Sector New England and CompassPoint Nonprofit Services, 2009), online at http://tsne.org/creative-disruption, on sabbaticals and nonprofits; see also Dan Wilford, "CEO Sabbatical: Prescription for a Healthier Organization," *Trustee: The Journal for Hospital Governing Boards* 45:7 (July 1992), 18–23; Vanessa Small, "Sabbatical Recharges Nonprofit CEO," *Washington Post* (20 May 2012), online at https:// www.washingtonpost.com/business/capitalbusiness/sabbatical-recharges -nonprofit-ceo/2012/05/18/gIQAhjlVdU_story.html.

Tarun Khanna, Jaeyong Song, and Kyungmook Lee, "The Paradox of Samsung's Rise," *Harvard Business Review* (July–August 2011), 142–147, and Verne Harnish, *The Greatest Business Decisions of All Time* (New York: Liberty Street, 2012), discuss Samsung's sabbatical program.

Josiah Bunting III, "Gen. George C. Marshall and the Development of a Professional Military Ethic," *Foreign Policy Research Institute Footnotes* 16:4 (June 2011), 1–5, is the main source for my discussion of US generals between the wars; see also D. K. R. Crosswell, *Beetle: The Life of General Walter Bedell Smith* (Lexington: University Press of Kentucky, 2010); Jean Edward Smith, *Lucius D. Clay: An American Life* (New York: Henry Holt & Company, 1990).

Henry Lowood, "Douglas Engelbart Interview 1," 19 December 1986, Stanford University Library, http://web.stanford.edu/dept/SUL /library/prod//depts/hasrg/histsci/ssvoral/engelbart/engfmst1-ntb.html, has Engelbart's description of his time on Leyte; see also Thierry Bardini, *Bootstrapping: Douglas Engelbart, Coevolution, and the Origins of Personal Computing* (Stanford, CA: Stanford University Press, 2000), and Alexis Madrigal, "The Hut Where the Internet Began," *The Atlantic* (7 July 2013), online at http://www.theatlantic.com/technology/archive /2013/07/the-hut-where-the-internet-began/277551/. Penfield describes his sabbaticals in his autobiography, *No Man Alone*; he also describes working with Ramón y Cajal in *The Second Career*, esp. 82–85. My account of Lovelock draws on James Lovelock's autobiography, *Homage to Gaia: The Life of an Independent Scientist* (Oxford, UK: Oxford University Press, 2001), and James Lovelock's oral history with Paul Merchant, part of the British Library's National Life Stories Project, C1379/15, http:// sounds.bl.uk/related-content/TRANSCRIPTS/021T-C1379X0015XX -0000A1.pdf. Graham Wallas describes his 1923 trip in letters to his wife Ada, in the Wallas Family Papers, File 1/1/28, Newnham College, Cambridge; quotes are from Graham Wallas to Ada Wallas, 14 June 1923, 28 June 1923, and 18 June 1923.

Carmit T. Tadmor, Adam D. Galinsky, and William W. Maddux, "Getting the Most Out of Living Abroad: Biculturalism and Integrative Complexity as Key Drivers of Creative and Professional Success," *Journal of Personality and Social Psychology* 103:3 (2013), 520–542, is the source of the quote on biculturalism, on 520; see also: William W. Maddux and Adam D. Galinsky, "Cultural Borders and Mental Barriers: The Relationship Between Living Abroad and Creativity," *Journal of Personality and Social Psychology* 95 (2009), 1047–1061; William W. Maddux, Hajo Adam, and Adam D. Galinsky, "When in Rome . . . Learn Why the Romans Do What They Do: How Multicultural Learning Experiences Facilitate Creativity," *Personality and Social Psychology Bulletin* 36 (2010), 731–741; Jiyin Cao, Adam D. Galinsky, and William W. Maddux, "Does Travel Broaden the Mind?: Breadth of Foreign Experiences Increases

Generalized Trust," *Social Psychological and Personality Science* 5:5 (July 2014), 517–525; Frédéric C. Godart et al., "Fashion with a Foreign Flair: Professional Experiences Abroad Facilitate the Creative Innovations of Organizations," *Academy of Management Journal* 58:1 (February 2015), 195–220. Angela Ka-yee Leung et al., "Multicultural Experience Enhances Creativity: The When and How," *American Psychologist* 63 (2008), 169–181, provides an overview of Adam Galinsky's work on travel, biculturalism, and creativity.

See Oranit B. Davidson, et al., "Sabbatical Leave: Who Gains and How Much?," *Journal of Applied Psychology* 95:5 (2010), 953–964, on detachment and academic sabbaticals.

Conclusion

Annie Dillard contrasts days and lives reading in *The Writing Life* (New York: Harper Perennial, 2013), 33; Spencer's observations on Lubbock are from Herbert Spencer, *An Autobiography* (London: Williams and Norgate, 1904), 72–3; Sun Tzu's advice is described in Thomas Cleary, "Translator's Introduction," in Sun Tzu, *The Art of War* (Boulder, CO: Shambhala Publications, 1988), xviii; Miyamoto Musashi, *The Book of Five Rings* (Radford, CA: Wilder Publications, 2008), 30; William James, "Gospel of Relaxation," in *On Vital Reserves: The Energies of Men; The Gospel of Relaxation* (New York: Henry Holt, 1911), 61.

William Davies, *The Happiness Industry: How the Government and Big Business Sold Us Well-Being* (London: Verso Books, 2015) discusses how businesses try to convert passion into corporate assets. Eiduson's study is described in Robert S. Root-Bernstein, Maurine Bernstein, and Helen Garnier, "Correlations Between Avocations, Scientific Style, Work Habits, and Professional Impact of Scientists."

Penfield, *The Second Career*, 186; Osler, "The Practitioner of Medicine," in Osler, *Counsels and Ideals* (Oxford, UK: Henry Frowde, 1905), 196–197; Osler, "Work," in *Counsels and Ideals*, 236; John Lubbock, "Recreation," in *The Use of Life* (London: Macmillan and Co., 1895), 69.

Index